Venous disease
SIMPLIFIED

T0178853

Edited by
Alun H Davies, Tim A Lees & Ian F Lane

tfm Publishing Limited, Castle Hill Barns, Harley, Nr Shrewsbury, SY5 6LX, UK

Tel: +44 (0)1952 510061; Fax: +44 (0)1952 510192
E-mail: nikki@tfmpublishing.com; Web site: www.tfmpublishing.com

Design: Nikki Bramhill, tfm publishing Ltd.
Typesetting: Nikki Bramhill, tfm publishing Ltd.
First Edition: June 2006

ISBN 1 903378 25 7

Printed by Gutenberg Press Ltd., Gudja Road, Tarxien, PLA 19, Malta. Tel: +356 21897037; Fax: +356 21800069.

Contents

Contributors

Andrew W Bradbury BSc MD MBA FRCS (Ed) Professor of Vascular Surgery, Birmingham University Department of Vascular Surgery, Heart of England NHS Foundation Trust, Birmingham, UK

Kevin Burnand MS FRCS Professor in Surgery, Head of the Academic Department of Surgery, St. Thomas' Hospital, London, UK

Joseph A Caprini MD MS FACS RVT Louis W. Biegler Professor of Surgery and Bioengineering, Department of Surgery, Evanston Northwestern Healthcare, Evanston, Illinois, USA; Northwestern University Feinberg School of Medicine, Chicago, Illinois, USA and Robert R. McCormick School of Engineering and Applied Sciences, Evanston, Illinois, USA

Katy AL Darvall MB ChB MRCS (Eng) Research Fellow, Birmingham University Department of Vascular Surgery, Heart of England NHS Foundation Trust, Birmingham, UK

Alun H Davies MA (Cantab & Oxon) DM (Oxon) FRCS Reader in Surgery and Consultant Surgeon, Imperial College School of Medicine, Charing Cross Hospital, London, UK

Linda de Cossart ChM FRCS Consultant Vascular and General Surgeon, Countess of Chester NHS Foundation Trust, Chester, UK

Jonothan J Earnshaw DM FRCS Consultant Surgeon, Gloucestershire Royal Hospital, Gloucester, UK

Gerry Fowkes PhD FRCPE FFPH Professor of Epidemiology/Director of Wolfson Unit for Prevention of Peripheral Vascular Diseases, University of Edinburgh, Edinburgh, Scotland

Manj Gohel MRCS Vascular Research Fellow, Cheltenham General Hospital, Cheltenham, UK

Monica D Hansrani MD MB BS FRCS Specialist Registrar, Northern Vascular Centre, Freeman Hospital, Newcastle upon Tyne, UK

Ian F Lane MA DM MCh FRCS Consultant Vascular Surgeon, University Hospital of Wales, Cardiff, UK

Tim A Lees MB ChB FRCS MD Consultant Vascular Surgeon, Northern Vascular Centre, Freeman Hospital, Newcastle upon Tyne, UK

Keith Poskitt MD FRCS Consultant Surgeon, Cheltenham General Hospital, Cheltenham, UK

Nung Rudarakanchana MA MB BChir PhD (Cantab) House Officer, Charing Cross Hospital, London, UK

Rachel C Sam MA MB ChB MRCS (Eng) Specialist Registrar, Birmingham University Department of Vascular Surgery, Heart of England NHS Foundation Trust, Birmingham, UK

John H Scurr BSc MB BS FRCS Consultant Surgeon, The Lister Hospital, London, UK

Beverley Sharp MB BS BSc MRCS AKC Clinical Fellow, Charing Cross Hospital, London, UK

Fiona Slim RGN Senior Surgical Care Practitioner, Cheltenham General Hospital, Cheltenham, UK

Philip Coleridge Smith DM FRCS Reader in Surgery, UCL Medical School, London, UK

Gerard Stansby MChir MB FRCS Professor of Vascular Surgery, Northern Vascular Centre, Freeman Hospital, Newcastle upon Tyne, UK

Justin Tan MRCS Clinical Research Fellow, St. Thomas' Hospital, London, UK

Maxine Taylor BSc (Hons) RGN Senior Leg Ulcer Nurse Specialist, Cheltenham General Hospital, Cheltenham, UK

Marianne Vandendriessche MD FRCS (Belg) Consultant Vascular Surgeon, Jan Palfyn Hospital, Gent, Belgium and London Vein Institute, UK

Mark Whiteley MS FRCS (Gen) FRCS (Ed) MB BS Consultant Vascular Surgeon, The Whiteley Clinic, Guildford, UK

Mark Whyman MS FRCS Consultant Surgeon, Cheltenham General Hospital, Cheltenham, UK

Preface

The management of venous disease is going through a period of rapid development with the appearance of several new non-invasive treatments, including laser ablation, radiofrequency ablation and foam sclerotherapy. Nevertheless, other modalitities of treatment developed many years ago have stood the test of time and are still in use today.

This book aims to produce a balanced up-to-date view of the management of venous disease, from the simplest cutaneous thread veins to complex chronic venous insufficiency and deep venous thrombosis. We are grateful for the contributions of many established experts in the field of venous disease, who have shared their knowledge and experience of managing a variety of venous conditions.

Each chapter concludes with a list of summary points and references. We hope that the reader will enjoy the text and that it will improve their understanding of venous problems.

We are also grateful to Nikki Bramhill of tfm Publishing who has worked tirelessly to produce a well structured book in record time.

Alun H Davies
Tim A Lees
Ian F Lane

Chapter 1
The history and importance of venous disease in modern practice

Ian F Lane MA DM MCh FRCS

Consultant Vascular Surgeon, University Hospital of Wales, Cardiff, UK

Introduction

The modern management of venous disease is inextricably linked with advances in physiological measurement and imaging. Indeed, early accounts of disorders describe anomalies and only in the mid-20th century was there an attempt to merge 'form and function'. Varicose veins have been reported for thousands of years with one of the earliest accounts of serpent-shaped dilatation of the lower limbs from about 1552BC in the Ebers papyrus (Figure 1). The first reliable description of intervention for extremity varices appears in a Turkish textbook, *Imperial Surgery*, written in 1465AD, although procedures appear to have taken place during the earlier Byzantine period. A published case history of venous thrombosis is recognised at the Bibliothèque Nationale in Paris, affecting a Normandy man aged 20 years in 1282AD. The patient sustained unilateral oedema with ulceration and exudation, and although able to walk only with crutches initially, the symptoms eventually settled leaving only mild long-term leg throbbing. Probably the most significant early work was by Fabricus in 1603 and his student

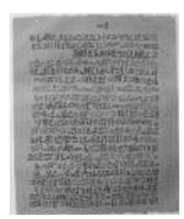

Figure 1 The Ebers papyrus was discovered in Egypt in the 1870s and contains 877 recipes for diseases or symptoms.

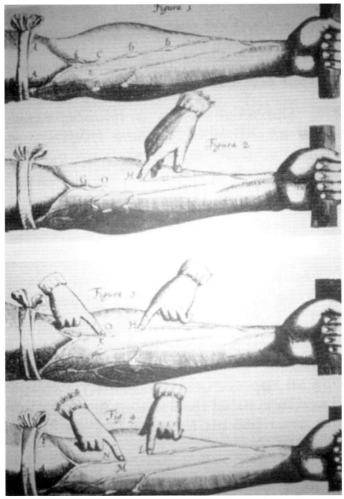

Figure 2 Illustration of venous valves from Harvey's 1628 book *De Moto Cordis*.

Harvey in 1628, who described the structure and function of venous valves and the circulatory system respectively (Figure 2).

Paré in the 16th century underpinned surgical principles and these were developed by Trendelenburg (Figure 3) and others around the

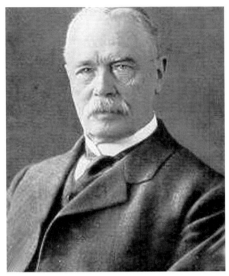

Figure 3 Friedrick Trendelenburg (1844-1924) was Surgeon-in-Chief at Leipzig.
Courtesy of www.historiadelamedicina.org.

beginning of the 20th century, leading to Keller and Mayo in 1905/6 performing the first ablation of the great saphenous vein, thus providing a gateway to the modern era [1, 2].

Historical landmarks

Investigation of venous disorders

Clinical examination with use of the Trendelenberg test and tourniquet has been the mainstay of diagnosis of superficial venous incompetence, even in recent years, despite the inaccuracies in differentiation of saphenopopliteal and perforator disease. The recognition of the physiological implications of deep venous incompetence remained elusive until the era of pulsed Doppler ultrasound imaging and flow measurements. Plethysmography was developed in the mid-20th century

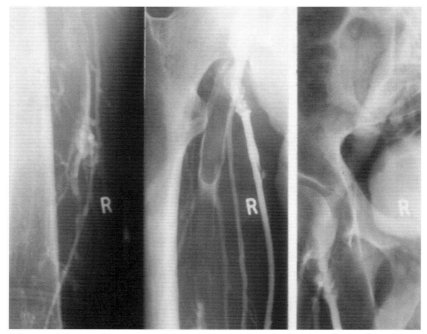

Figure 4 Ascending venogram with thrombus in the femoral vein.

and is based upon measurment of venous refill times using strain gauge, electrical impedance or skin colour changes. Difficulties with reproducibility and standardisation has meant that plethysmography has limited use in clinical practice but is valuable in venous research, particularly where continual assessment of individual patients is required.

Contrast venography was popularised in the 1960s and even now is regarded by many as the gold standard for the diagnosis of deep vein thrombosis (Figure 4). Descending femoral venography enabled diagnosis of deep venous incompetence based upon distal reflux of contrast, although the clinical implications of single or multiple valvular reflux are not clear. Venography or phlebography is still of value in planning surgery for pelvic venous obstruction and determining the origin of atypical lower limb varicosities, but its use has largely been superseded by duplex imaging.

Continuous-wave Doppler ultrasound has been used in fluid engineering since the 1950s and was further developed, initially in arterial disease where the velocity shifts are significant, by Satomura in the 1970s, when the importance of ankle/brachial systolic pressure indices was recognised. Strandness popularised the technique in both arterial and venous disease, but now modern duplex ultrasound systems combine flow measurement with imaging, enabling the function of individual valves to be identified whilst examining the quality of vein wall, as well as identifying deep vein thrombosis [3]. The accurate assessment of perforator and pelvic vein incompetence has led to dilemmas in the significance, and need for treatment, of these conditions. Initial early concerns over the size of ultrasound equipment have been addressed by development of portable devices, although considerable operator training and experience is required. Hand-held Dopper devices, measuring flow alone, are useful as an adjunct to clinical examination but have limited specificity in determining saphenopopliteal and deep vein incompetence. Both duplex imaging and Doppler flow assessment have ensured that surgery for venous incompetence can be planned and is appropriate with venous surgeons recommending that all patients undergo pre-operative investigation.

Modern imaging techniques such as CT angiography have found a place in the diagnosis of pulmonary emboli, whilst magnetic resonance venography may be useful in the management of pelvic and thoracic outlet venous obstruction in the future.

Sclerotherapy and other local treatments

Sclerotherapy was commenced by Pravaz in approximately 1860 and promoted in Europe in 1947 with the foundation of Sociètè Francaise de Phlebologie. Fegan subsequently popularised and developed the technique that bears his name, although by the late 20th century enthusiasm, certainly in the UK, was reducing [4]. The reasons for this were the recognition that sclerotherapy did not address the underlying valvular incompetence, leading to high recurrence rates reported as 90% at ten years, patient acceptability of prolonged compression and complications of the technique including ulceration and skin staining. Recently, the development of less toxic intravenous agents and the introduction of foam sclerotherapy under duplex guidance has led to a renaissance of the procedure. Foaming of the sclerosant enables the injection to remain within the targeted vein and can be accurately followed to the saphenofemoral junction. Trials of the technique are underway but if long-term recurrence rates are low then traditional surgery will be challenged. Within Europe the practice of phlebology is widespread leading to a new specialty for venous disease that is not found in the UK.

The rise in demand for cosmetic surgery has led to increasing requests for treatment of telangiectasia or 'spider veins'. These are mainly present on the legs and can be unsightly, but normally are asymptomatic. A number of techniques are available including fine needle sclerotherapy using loupes and a 30-gauge needle, photodynamic therapy and laser. The result is not predictable on an individual basis and recurrence is usual as this is a progressive disease.

Surgery for varicose veins

Trendelenberg in 1891, described ligation of the great saphenous vein in the mid-thigh as a treatment for varicose veins, but the significance of flush saphenofemoral ligation was not appreciated until 1904 when Tavel indicated the advisability of this procedure in order to prevent recurrence. It was not until 1906 that Keller and Mayo described stripping with the operative techniques refined by Turner Warwick in the 1930s. Linton at same time published an account of the classic subfascial ligation of the perforating veins with a revival by Cockett in 1953 who applied a similar technique to the treatment of venous ulcers [5]. The problems of operating through the infected ulcer base to ligate the perforators has been overcome with the recent development of Subfascial Endoscopic Perforator Ligation (SEPS) but even so, the procedure remains controversial with much debate over the significance of incompetence at this site (Figure 5).

Contrast imaging initially confirmed the importance of flush ligation of incompetent valves in order to prevent recurrence, but duplex ultrasound now ensures that visualisation is both sensitive and non-invasive. Latterly,

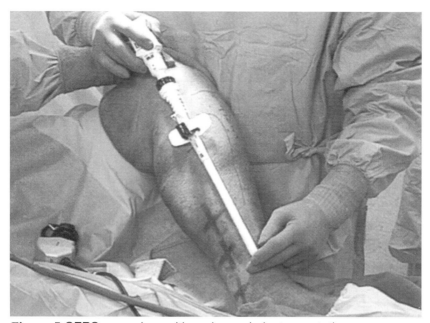

Figure 5 SEPS procedure with endoscopic instrumentation.

not only is the need to treat Hunterian thigh perforators and the Giacomini vein recognised, but vulval varicosities, pelvic tributaries and other minor branch incompetencies have been identified, posing dilemmas as to the need for ligation which are still debated today. The 1980s were concerned with the prevention of recurrence after saphenofemoral ligation. Initially all recurrence was attributed to incorrect surgery and inability to ligate all branches of the saphenofemoral junction, particularly when the majority of varicose vein surgery at that time was performed by trainees. Controlled trials, following up patients in whom duplex imaging immediately after surgery revelealed complete saphenofemoral ligation, indicated that neovascularisation was the cause of recurrence in many cases. Attempts to prevent this regrowth of veins with formal closure of the cribriform fascia, Dacron patch interposition between the closed saphenofemoral junction and superficial tissues, and diathermy obliteration of the endothelium of the exposed vein stump have not been universally accepted into surgical practice.

Despite the technique being over 100 years old, stripping of the great saphenous vein continues to be popular and effective. Concerns over pain and morbidity, particularly with much surgery now performed as a day case, has led to refinements to the original steel Babcock instrument, which pleated the vein on an acorn-shaped head. The introduction of PIN stripping and perforation-invagination removal of the great saphenous vein is gaining popularity. Avoidance of stripping with removal of the great saphenous vein by sequential avulsions, although described, has not gained enthusiastic support. The risk of damage to the saphenous nerve during stripping was recognised in the 1960s and can be avoided by not progressing below the upper third of the calf, although the nerve can still be traumatised by calf avulsions. Flush saphenofemoral ligation without removal of the great saphenous vein was popularised in the 1980s with encouraging short-term results. Although the technique theoretically may preserve a great saphenous vein for later coronary artery bypass surgery, prolonged follow-up showed unacceptable recurrence rates and the procedure has now largely been abandoned.

Contemporary innovative techniques now allow a surgeon and ultrasonographer to work together and accurately identify the saphenofemoral junction allowing obliteration of the vein by intraluminally applied laser or local heat. Modern engineering technology has enabled these advances, although the use of intraluminal diathermy to destroy the vein was described in the 1970s. The branches of the great saphenous vein can subsequently be obliterated by sclerotherapy and whilst the whole procedure is available under local anaesthesia, the long-term recurrence rate is as yet unknown.

Venous ulcers, deep vein thrombosis and venous reconstruction

Historically, lower limb ulcers have been a curiosity and well described, but their aetiology cannot be confirmed as venous. An association between ulceration and the absence of varicose veins was recognised by Gay and Spender as early as 1868. However, it was ascending and descending venography that identified the likely cause of venous ulcers as deep vein obstruction or incompetence, leading to calf muscle pump dysfunction. The use of resting and ambulatory intraluminal venous pressure measurement as a research tool indicated, in the 1960s, the physiological abnormality, although the pathological process at cellular level still remains uncertain. Calf perforator incompetence has been considered as an aetiological factor for ulceration. Perforator ligation, initially promoted by Linton in 1938 and subsequently performed either subfascially via a 'stocking seam' incision or extrafascially through the ulcer base, remained difficult to assess, as the accompanying prolonged bed rest was known to promote ulcer healing. Indeed the early part of the latter 20th century was characterised by many patients with venous ulcers remaining in hospital beds with their legs elevated for many weeks. Ulcer healing was generally assured but there was often breakdown of the skin within days of returning home.

The pathology of the tissue death has been subject to considerable cell biology and pharmaceutical research. The 1970s were concerned over a finding that a pericapillary fibrin cuff could impair oxygen diffusion leading to ulceration. The fibrinolytic and anabolic steroid, stanozolol, was used as treatment but eventually abandoned due to insufficient evidence of efficacy and unwanted androgenic effect [6]. A little later the observation that leucocytes accumulated in dependent ulcerated legs led to the hypothesis that plugging of capillaries leading to local ischaemia may occur.

Modern treatment of venous ulcers involves excluding other causes such as arterial or auto-immune disease, correction of any venous abnormality and community care with regular use of compression bandages and hosiery when epithelialisation takes place. Elastic stockings were described by Taberer in Nottingham in the 1840s, although Wiseman is said to have made leather supportive stockings in 1676. Their design has been refined with the compression forces at the ankle now subject to international standardisation. The measurement of venous filling times by plethysmography and tourniquet can apportion the relative contribution between deep and superficial incompetence, although superficial surgery needs to be performed with caution and the results are unpredictable. Repair of incompetant valves, either by transplantation from the arm or surrounding with a Dacron sling, is still experimental, although early results

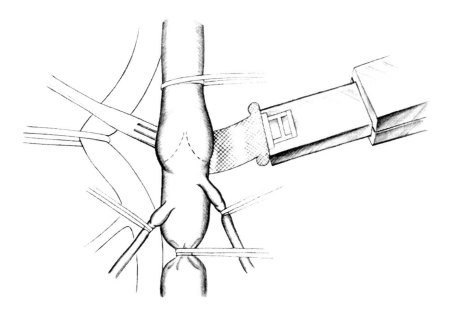

Figure 6 Sling repair of an incompetent valve.

from Australia in the 1980s were encouraging (Figure 6). Patients for valve reconstruction need to be selected with care, as post-thrombotic disease with a thickened vein wall is unsuitable for surgery, leaving only a small cohort with constitutional deep vein incompetence.

Venous thrombosis and associated pulmonary emboli were recognised by Virchow in 1846 and his triad of hypercoagulability, stasis and vessel wall damage as a cause remains appropriate today. There have been many advances in the diagnosis of deep vein thrombosis since initial contrast venography but anticoagulation remains the basis for prevention of recurrence. Venous thrombectomy for deep vein thrombosis, introduced in 1938 and now rarely performed, was complicated by early rethrombosis, due to the intense inflammatory reaction in the vein wall. Prevention of pulmonary emboli by femoral vein ligation was suggested by Homans in 1934 but was associated with lower limb complications and a 5% to 8% rate of fatal recurrent embolism. Further techniques involved either complete or partial occlusion of the inferior vena cava by sutures or clips, but it was not until the advent of the Mobin-Uddin umbrella catheter in 1969 that a practical method of caval interruption was available, leading to further development of percutaneous filters. Unfortunately, patency rates of venous bypass procedures for obstruction do not compare with arterial reconstruction success. The classic Palma operation for unilateral iliac vein obstruction was introduced in Uruguay in 1958 and requires a pressure gradient between both femoral veins to maintain patency of the graft. The long-term results are poor and it seems likely, in the absence of an effective prosthetic vein graft, that the major advances in relief of venous obstruction will be through balloon dilatation and intraluminal stenting.

Conclusions

The prevalence of varicose veins has been estimated at 2% of the population with the treatment of venous ulcers costing approximately 0.5% of the National Health Service budget. The need for both anatomical and physiological recognition of abnormality in order to plan treatment is now understood. The last 20 years have seen a resurgence of science into venous disorders and formation of national professional societies of physicians, nurses and technicians in Europe and the USA. Treatment of varicose veins is likely to take place outside the traditional hospital environment using minimally invasive ultrasound-assisted techniques avoiding general anaesthesia. There will be increasing discussion over cost-benefit analysis, complications and changes in quality of life, although demand will be patient led. Ultimately, procedures will be dependent upon modern technology, but the cure of deep venous incompetence still remains elusive.

Key Summary

◆ Venous disease has been recorded for over 2000 years.

◆ Contrast venography remained a gold standard for much of the 20th century.

◆ Duplex imaging has advanced knowledge of physiology.

◆ Future interventional developments will be led by technology.

◆ Management of deep venous insufficiency remains challenging.

References

1. Browse NL, Burnand KG, Lea Thomas M. *Diseases of Veins*. London: Edward Arnold, 1988.
2. Bernstein M, Koo HP, Bloom DA. Beyond the Trendelenburg position: Friedrich Trendelenburg's life and surgical contributions. *Surgery, St Louis* 1999; 126(1): 78-82.
3. Bergan JJ. Historical highlights in treating venous insufficiency. In: *Venous Disorders*. Bergan JJ, Yao JST, Eds. Philadelphia: WB Saunders, 1991: 3-15.
4. Fegan G. *Varicose Veins: Compression Sclerotherapy*. London: Heinemann Medical, 1967.
5. Linton RR. The communicating veins of the lower leg and the operative technic for their ligation. *Ann Surg* 1938; 107(4): 582-93.
6. Browse NL, Burnand KG. The cause of venous ulceration. *Lancet* 1982; 243-5.

Chapter 2

Epidemiology of venous disease

Gerry Fowkes PhD FRCPE FFPH

*Professor of Epidemiology/Director of Wolfson Unit for Prevention of Peripheral
Vascular Diseases, University of Edinburgh, Edinburgh, Scotland*

Introduction

Venous disease in the legs is commonplace and may present in many
different ways. Conditions include: classic varicose veins (trunk varices);
minor varices such as telangiectasia and reticular varices; and chronic
venous insufficiency which may comprise skin changes including
ulceration. These conditions are considered to be linked aetiologically and
on a spectrum of severity. In this chapter, the frequency of occurrence of
these conditions in the community will be described and the risk factors
which may be important in causation will be discussed. Also, the
epidemiology of deep vein thrombosis, a condition also covered in
Chapter 12, will be described briefly.

Given the different categories of venous disease, and the varieties of
presentation and severity, there has over the years been some confusion
around terminology and definition of venous diseases. This has led to
considerable difficulties, particularly in epidemiological research in which
it is important to have standard definitions for comparisons between
studies and of disease over time, either in the individual or in the
population. For this reason, attempts have been made to develop standard
classifications and of these the most widely accepted is CEAP (Clinical-
Etiology-Anatomy-Pathophysiology) [1]. This classification is being
constantly updated as new knowledge becomes available. The latest
version of the clinical classification is shown in Table 1.

Table 1 The latest version of the CEAP (Clinical-Etiology-Anatomy-Pathophysiology) classification.

C_0	No visible or palpable signs of venous disease
C_1	Telangiectasia or reticular veins
C_2	Varicose veins (distinguished from reticular veins by diameter of 3mm or more)
C_3	Oedema
C_4	Changes in skin and subcutaneous tissue secondary to chronic venous disease
C_{4a}	Pigmentation or eczema
C_{4b}	Lipodermatosclerosis or atrophie blanche
C_5	Healed venous ulcer
C_6	Active venous ulcer

Unfortunately, most epidemiological research on venous disease was carried out before development of the CEAP system, and this may be one reason why there is considerable discrepancy between the results found in different studies.

Frequency of venous disease in the general population

In epidemiological studies, the frequency of disease is normally described in two ways:

◆ the prevalence rate which is the proportion of the whole population who have the disease at a defined point or period of time; and
◆ the incidence rate which is the proportion of individuals free of disease who acquire it over a defined length of time.

Finding out the prevalence of disease requires a survey of the whole population, or a sample, at one point in time, whereas finding out the incidence rate requires that a population free of the disease are followed-up over a length of time, often many years, to ascertain who acquires the disease. Thus, prevalence studies (cross-sectional surveys) are usually much easier to carry out than incidence studies (cohort studies), and so more evidence is available on the prevalence than the incidence of disease.

Asymptomatic venous disease (CEAP C_0)

In venous disease, a key underlying pathogenic factor is incompetence of venous valves. However, such incompetence resulting in valvular reflux may occur in individuals without signs or symptoms of venous disease.

The advent in recent years of duplex scanning has permitted vein reflux to be measured non-invasively in epidemiological studies. One of the few studies to carry out duplex scanning was the Edinburgh Vein Study [2], in which a random sample of men and women in the general population aged 18 to 64 years were scanned. Around 35% of subjects without overt evidence of venous disease had significant reflux ($\geq$0.5 seconds) in at least one of eight venous segments measured in each leg. Thus, venous insufficiency in the legs may occur with no evidence of varicose veins or other clinical manifestation. The Bochum studies [3] in Germany have demonstrated that such reflux may occur in the teenage years when it is much more common than clinical varicosities. For example, among 14-16-year-olds examined in the Bochum Study II, 12.3% had saphenous reflux, but only 1.7% had trunk varices, 0.8% had tributary varices and 4.1% incompetent perforators.

Telangiectasia and reticular varices (CEAP C_1)

The population prevalences of minor categories of varicose veins, such as telangiectasia and reticular varices, are difficult to determine because most studies do not provide such information, and the classification of the categories and their severity varies between studies. In the Basle Study [4] of workers in the pharmaceutical industry, 5.2% of men and 3.2% of women were considered to have trunk varices, but a much higher proportion (51.8% of men and 64.8% of women) had reticular varices and/or telangiectasia. In the Edinburgh Vein Study, both reticular varices and telangiectasia were found in over 80% of subjects, although most were relatively mild (Figure 1). Clearly, more information is required on the

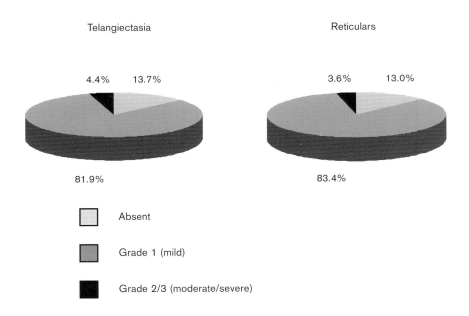

Telangiectasia

4.4%   13.7%

81.9%

Reticulars

3.6%   13.0%

83.4%

☐ Absent

▨ Grade 1 (mild)

■ Grade 2/3 (moderate/severe)

Figure 1 Prevalence of telangiectasia and reticular varices in the Edinburgh Vein Study (adjusted for age and sex).

frequency of telangiectasia and reticular varices, and also the extent to which they are linked to current or future occurrence of trunk varicose veins.

Trunk varicose veins (CEAP C_2)

Since the 1960s many surveys have been carried out in different countries investigating the frequency of classic trunk (stem) varicose veins. However, differences in the populations studied and the definitions and methods of recruiting patients make comparisons difficult and, indeed, wildly different results have been obtained from different surveys. Nevertheless, a reasonable estimate of the prevalence of varicose veins in western populations can be obtained from studies based on general population samples, mainly in the USA and Europe. Although the definitions of disease and methods of measurement were slightly different between studies, the prevalence of varicose veins in females was remarkably consistent with around one quarter to one third of women affected. There is also little doubt from the majority of epidemiological studies that a higher prevalence of varicose veins has been observed in females than in males. Prevalences derived from earlier surveys in the general population suggest that the female:male ratio was approximately 2:1. This male:female difference has also been shown in some later surveys, but in the Edinburgh Vein Study [2] a slightly higher prevalence was found in men, and this was also noted in young adults in the Bochum Study [3] in Germany. These are recent studies and there is a possibility that the prevalence of varicose veins may be increasing in men. Also, the higher prevalence in women in some studies may have been due partly to recruitment bias, because relatively more women were concerned about the cosmetic appearance of their varicosities and volunteered to take part.

A universal finding in epidemiological studies is that the prevalence of varicose veins increases with age. For example, in men in the Edinburgh Vein Study [2], prevalence increased from around 16% in those aged 25-34 years to 61% in those 55-64 years. For women aged 25-34 years, prevalence was 14% rising to 51% in those 55-64 years of age. In the Bochum Study [3], examination of schoolchildren aged 10-12 years demonstrated the presence of only discrete reticular varices in 10% of the pupils, but four years later this figure had increased to 30%, and a few children had developed stem and branch varices.

There has been much anecdotal evidence over the years that varicose veins are rare in developing countries, such as in Africa, compared to western countries. Meaningful comparisons between countries, however, can only be made if studies use the same methods and are based on population surveys. In this regard, a study investigating varicose veins in New Zealand and the South Pacific [5] is of interest because any differences were more likely to be real than to be due to methodological biases. Figure 2 shows that a marked difference in prevalence was found between the populations; for example, 44% of New Zealand Maori women had varicose veins compared to less than 5% of Atoll islanders. Furthermore, the prevalence among the New Zealand Maoris was similar to that of New Zealand caucasians. More recently in Southern California,

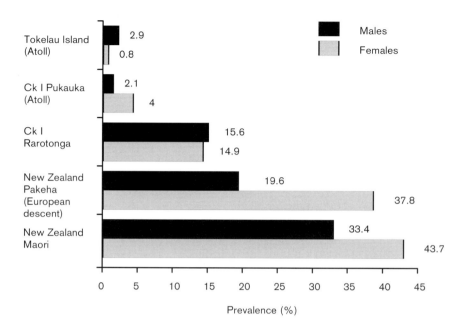

Figure 2 Prevalence (%) of varicose veins by sex in New Zealand and South Pacific Islands [5].

no differences were found in the prevalence of trunk varices between caucasian, hispanic, black and asian Americans [6]. These results are suggestive that varicose veins may occur less frequently in developing countries but on adopting more western lifestyles, within developed countries, the prevalence becomes similar between ethnic groups.

Although there have been many studies examining the prevalence of varicose veins, very little data are available on the incidence, that is the rate of development of new cases. In the Framingham Study [7], the annual incidence was found to be 1.9% per annum in men and 2.6% in women. Interestingly, the incidence did not increase with age so that the observed increase in the prevalence of varicose veins would appear to have been a result of the relatively constant development of cases as people grew older. Thus, increasing age *per se* would not appear to be a risk factor for the development of varicose veins.

Skin changes of chronic venous insufficiency (CEAP C_3, C_4)

The prevalence in the general population of skin changes due to venous insufficiency, such as hyperpigmentation, eczema and oedema, have not been well documented. In a population study in Tecumseh, USA [8], 3.7% of women and 3.0% of men had evidence of skin changes. The prevalence increased markedly with age so that, for example, in women, only 1.8% of those aged 30-39 years had skin changes compared to 20.7% of those over 70 years of age. In the Basle Study [4], the prevalence of 'pronounced' skin changes (dilatation of subcutaneous veins, hyper or hypopigmentation) was found in 9.6% of women and 8.7% of the men. Mild skin changes in the form of a venous flare occurred in 15% of women and 10% of men. These results were, however, based on active chemical industry employees and not on the general population. Nevertheless, the results from both the Basle and Tecumseh studies suggest that there is not such a large female to male preponderance of skin changes as there is for varicose veins.

In surveys of individuals with varicose veins, a considerable proportion have evidence of skin changes. For example, in a survey of varicose vein patients in Brazil [9], oedema was the commonest manifestation occurring in nearly 20% of subjects, while hyperpigmentation occurred in 6% and eczema in 1-2%. Likewise, the community-based study in Tecumseh, USA [8], found that 10% of men and 20% of women with varicose veins had oedema. The prevalence and severity of various grades of skin change were shown in the Basle Study [4] to relate to the severity of varicose veins. Among those with severe varicose veins (marked trunk varices), the prevalence of skin changes or ulceration was 81% and among those with minor varicose veins (reticular veins and/or telangiectasia or 'scarcely visible trunk varices') the prevalence was 30%. However, other than severity of varicosities, little is known about which varicose veins are at higher risk of acquiring skin changes.

Venous ulcers (CEAP C$_5$, C$_6$)

In epidemiological surveys, it is important to distinguish between the occurrence of open (active) ulcers in the population and the combination of open and healed ulcers, because very different figures will prevail. Overall, a very approximate estimate of the prevalence of open venous ulceration in the adult population over 18 years of age in western countries is about 0.3%. That is, about one in 350 adults are affected at any one time. For every patient with an open ulcer in the population, there would appear to be between two and four individuals with healed ulcers, so that the population prevalence of open and healed ulcers combined is around 1% [10, 11]. It would appear from epidemiological surveys that the prevalence of ulcers is around two to three times more common in females than males. Chronic leg ulceration is relatively uncommon below the age of 60 years. Above that, the prevalence increases consistently with age in both men and women [10, 11] with the female predominance being maintained at all ages.

The prognosis of chronic venous ulcers is often poor. Typically, in patients attending for treatment, only half the ulcers are healed within four months. In the Lothian and Forth Valley Leg Ulcer Study [10] carried out in the community in Scotland, more than 25% of ulcers had not healed after two years (Figure 3). The longest duration was 62 years in an 85-year-old woman. In a similar way the duration of the ulcer diathesis, i.e. the length of time in which ulcer patients in a community have experienced ulcers, irrespective of whether they were consistently open, has been investigated retrospectively. In the Lothian and Forth Valley Study [10], 45% had had episodes for more than ten years and 21% for between five and ten years. The number of episodes of active ulceration has also been investigated: approximately one third have been shown to have had one episode and at least another third to have had four or more episodes.

Deep vein thrombosis

Determining the frequency of deep vein thrombosis (DVT) in the community is difficult because DVT cannot be diagnosed solely by history and physical examination alone, but requires specialist investigation. Most of the evidence on incidence is available from the detection of cases

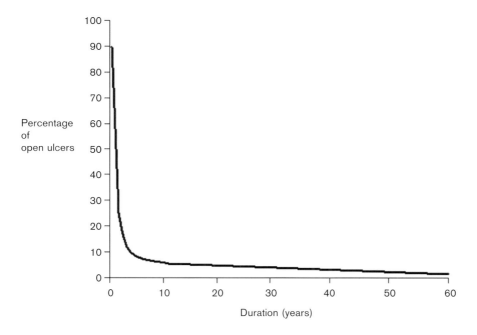

Figure 3 Duration of ulcers identified in the Lothian and Forth Valley Leg Ulcer Study in Scotland [10].

diagnosed in healthcare facilities serving a defined population. A systematic review has been carried out of such studies in order to provide a comprehensive estimate of the incidence of DVT in the general population [12]. This review found that of nine studies conducted between 1976 and 2000, the mean incidence of first DVT in the whole general population was 5.04 (95% CI 4.70, 5.38) per 10,000 person years. The incidence was similar in males and females and increased dramatically with age from about two to three per 10,000 person years at age 30-49 to 20 per 10,000 person years at age 70-79. Around 40% of cases of DVT were idiopathic. This review also confirmed that an additional 1-2 per 10,000 have a new DVT combined with pulmonary embolism.

The incidence of DVT is very strongly age-related and in the population as a whole, is comparable in men and women. Also, the increased risks of DVT within subgroups of the general population were substantial. For example, institutionalisation has been associated with an eight-fold increase in risk of DVT or pulmonary embolism, and this rose to around 20-fold if accompanied by surgery. Trauma has been associated with a 13-fold increase and malignancy with a five-fold increase in risk. The relative risks of thrombo-embolism among women using oral contraceptives or hormone replacement therapy is around two to four compared to non-users. Inherited or acquired thrombophilia, such as those associated with activated protein C resistance and Factor V Leiden mutation, may also increase risk very substantially.

Risk factors for venous disease in the general population

Varicose veins

Epidemiological investigations on risk factors for varicose veins have been limited almost exclusively to trunk varices, with very little information on telangiectasia or reticular varices. Numerous genetic, lifestyle, and physiological characteristics have been put forward as possible risk factors for the development of trunk varicose veins. Many of these factors, such as low-fibre diet and lack of exercise, are associated with 'westernisation' and have been suggested as possible explanations for the apparent geographical variation in the prevalence of varicose veins. Figure 4 shows risk factors which have been studied and how they might feasibly interact to increase the risk of varicosities. However, the evidence linking most of these factors to the development of varicose veins is extremely limited, particularly as there have been very few properly conducted epidemiological studies. In this section, emphasis will be given to those factors in which the evidence linking them to varicose veins is strongest, especially parity and weight.

Parity

In women, varicose veins are believed to often appear for the first time during pregnancy. However, pregnancy could merely be an exacerbating

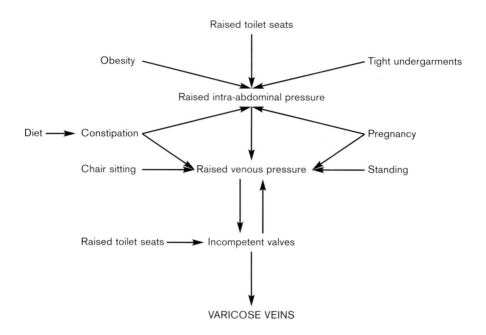

Figure 4 Possible interaction of genetic, cultural and physiological factors in the aetiology of varicose veins.

factor in those already predisposed, rather than a primary cause. Epidemiological studies have sought to determine whether a previous history of pregnancy or the number of pregnancies are related to the occurrence of varicose veins. In the population-based study in New Zealand and the South Pacific [5], a greater number of pregnancies in women of European origin was associated with an increasing prevalence of varicose veins, and in Maoris with a greater severity of varicose veins. The relationships between pregnancy and varicose veins was maintained on adjustment for age, height and weight. In a study with a more selected population in Brazil attending a health centre, a positive correlation was found between prevalence of varicose veins and number of previous pregnancies, independently of age [9].

In the Basle Study [4], age-adjusted rates of varicose veins were higher in multiparous than primiparous women, who in turn had higher rates than nulliparae. The Framingham Study [7] is the one longitudinal study to relate the incidence of varicose veins to various risk factors; it was found that the number of pregnancies was associated with incidence, although the association was statistically non-significant (p>0.05). The only population-based study which has not found a relationship with number of pregnancies was in Tecumseh, USA [8]. Nevertheless, the balance of the evidence at present would indicate that number of pregnancies is a risk factor for the development of varicose veins. The precise relative risks are difficult to determine, but results from the Basle and Framingham Studies [4, 7] indicate that women with two or more pregnancies, compared to those with a single pregnancy or no previous pregnancy, have an approximately 20% to 30% increased risk of developing varicose veins.

It is not clear why pregnancy might increase the risk of developing varicose veins. The common belief that pregnancy leads to varicose veins due to pressure of the pregnant uterus obstructing venous return from the legs has been refuted, because the majority of varices appear during the first three months of pregnancy when the uterus is not large enough to cause mechanical obstruction. A hormonal factor or the additional burden of increased circulating blood volume could be important.

Weight

Being overweight is commonly believed to be important in predisposing individuals to increased risk of varicose veins. In the Basle Study [4] of chemical workers in which the results were age-adjusted, varicose veins were more common in overweight women. But, in men, only telangiectasia and reticular varicosities, and not trunk varices, were more common in overweight individuals. In community surveys such as that in West Jerusalem, people with varicose veins have been shown to have a higher body mass index (kg/m^2) than normals [13]. In multivariate analyses including weight and height, weight remained significantly related to the occurrence of varicose veins in women, but not in men. Similarly, among caucasian New Zealanders, body mass index was related to severity of varicose veins only in women and independently of parity [5]. In the

Framingham Study [7], the incidence of varicose veins over a 16-year follow-up period was higher in subjects with a baseline body mass index of over $27kg/m^2$. On multivariate analysis the difference was maintained in women, but not in men. Thus, the balance of evidence, as confirmed in data from the Edinburgh Vein Study (Table 2) would suggest that a high body mass index is related to the occurrence of varicose veins, but the evidence is much more convincing for women than for men. It is also not clear whether the risk increases above a certain cut-off point or is apparent across the range of body mass index.

Table 2 Association between trunk varices and weight and body mass index in men and women in the Edinburgh Vein Study.

Trunk varices	Weight: kg	Body Mass Index: kg/m^2
Men		
None	79.18 (0.65)	25.79 (0.19)
Grade 1 (mild)	77.49 (0.77)	25.29 (0.25)
Grade 2 (moderate)	83.71 (2.11)	27.34 (0.73)
Grade 3 (severe)	79.60 (5.82)	26.43 (1.41)
p value for trend	NS	NS
Women		
None	65.72 (0.49)	25.06 (0.19)
Grade 1 (mild)	68.40 (0.89)	26.25 (0.35)
Grade 2 (moderate)	73.30 (2.14	27.44 (0.82)
Grade 3 (severe)	74.00 (11.82)	28.09 (3.23)
p value for trend	0.0001	0.0001

Values are mean (SE); NS = not significant

Standing and sitting

Prolonged standing has often been blamed for the development of varicose veins. Standing at work was shown to be positively associated with varicose veins in the study in Israel [13]. In the Framingham Study [7], the two-year incidence of varicose veins was higher with the length of time women spent sitting or standing but no significant difference was found relating posture to varicose veins in a study from Brazil [9]. Sitting in a chair has also been implicated. This practice is a western habit not adopted by primitive communities in which prevalence of varicose veins is apparently low. In New Guinea, varicose veins were common in men who sat with legs dangling, but rare in women who sat cross-legged on the ground, suggesting that variation in sitting positions might be the cause of this sex difference. Sitting in a chair could conceivably increase the hydrostatic pressure exerted on the leg veins, leading to pooling of blood in the legs, venous dilatation and increased tension in the wall itself. The effect of chair-sitting during childhood could therefore produce veins of an increased calibre which would be more susceptible to factors such as pregnancy, standing and tight clothes.

Bowel habit

The results of studies investigating bowel habit and varicose veins must often be interpreted with caution because of the difficulty of measuring constipation in a valid and reliable way. Among inhabitants of the South Pacific [5], the prevalence of varicose veins was low in primitive peoples, but high in more westernised cultures where the diet contained more refined carbohydrate and less dietary fibre. A typical low-fibre western diet produces small, hard stools which are difficult to pass, leading to regular straining and repeated increases in intra-abdominal pressure. In the Edinburgh Vein Study [2], straining in men was related to a higher risk of trunk varices. It has been postulated that during constipation, the loaded bowel compresses the iliac vein thus obstructing venous return from the legs, ultimately leading to the development of varicose veins. Alternatively, raised intra-abdominal pressure from straining may be transmitted down the veins of the legs, leading to dilation of the veins and non-apposition of the valve cusps, thus rendering the valves incompetent.

Many other factors have been implicated in the development of varicose veins. These include lack of exercise, cigarette smoking, and use of oral contraceptives. However, the evidence linking these and most of the other factors above to the occurrence of varicose veins is tenuous. The relationship between being overweight, parity and the occurrence of venous insufficiency is the most convincing, but for many factors, the relationship with varicose veins may be related more to confounding by other factors than a direct causal association. Evidence on the role of genetic predisposition in the development of varicose veins is limited and prone to considerable methodological difficulties, but this is an area of research ripe for development in order to identify new causative pathways of disease.

Venous ulcers

Severity of varicose veins

The risk of developing varicose ulcers would appear to increase with more severe varicose veins. In the Basle Study [4], for example, the risk of developing varicose ulcers during an 11-year follow-up period was 0.8% for those with mild varicosities, but 20% for those with severe varicose veins. There is also some evidence that the severity of venous incompetence, as indicated by objective measures such as the ambulatory venous pressure of the foot, may be related to the risk of ulceration.

Deep vein thrombosis

Deep vein thrombosis (DVT) is known to be an antecedent risk factor for the skin changes, oedema and ulceration associated with venous disease in the legs. Under these circumstances the venous condition is often referred to as the post-thrombotic syndrome. Although most studies do not separately identify ulcers or the number of ulcers are too small for meaningful analysis, the results linking DVT and the post-thrombotic syndrome are probably also meaningful in relation to ulcers alone.

In a population-based study of chronic venous ulcers in Perth, Western Australia [14], 17% of patients had a history of DVT and a large number had a history of conditions that might predispose to DVT. Although this prevalence seemed relatively high, results were unfortunately not available from a healthy comparison group. On the other hand, in a population-based study of 3,600 people in Copenhagen, Denmark [15], various risk factors were related to the occurrence of objective signs of venous disease. Previous thrombo-embolism (history of DVT or pulmonary embolism) was related to the occurrence of venous disease, independently of age, sex and other possible risk factors. The incidence of ulcers has been shown in follow-up studies of patients having a diagnosis of DVT to be around 1% to 2% per annum.

Arterial dsease

Arterial disease *per se* in the lower limbs is considered to be a cause of chronic leg ulceration, but the extent to which arterial disease might increase the risk of venous ulceration is less clear. Some studies have reported a relatively high prevalence of arterial disease in leg ulcer patients, but this may be partly accounted for by the presence of patients with ulcers primarily of arterial origin. Also, no comparisons were made with the occurrence of ulcers in a healthy control group. However, in a study based on the Lothian and Fourth Valley Leg Ulcer Study [10] in Scotland, arterial disease (angina, intermittent claudication, hypertension, and low ankle brachial pressure index) did not occur more commonly in 331 leg ulcer patients compared to an equal number of age- and sex-matched population controls.

Finally, several other factors may be possible contributory factors to the development of venous ulceration. These include minor trauma, oedema (not necessarily related to venous insufficiency), obesity, and coexisting conditions such as arthritis or neuropathies. However, the extent to which these factors are important is not well established, and are indicative of how little is known about the aetiology of venous disease.

Conclusions

The impact of venous disease on the community is considerable [16]. The morbidity associated with varicose veins is variable - leg symptoms such as heaviness, itching and cosmetic appearance dominate - and, overall, quality of life is diminished, although this is significantly improved following surgery. There is a huge demand for surgical treatment, much of which cannot be met: for example, 65,000 operations were performed on varicose veins in the UK in 1999. Venous ulcers are much more serious causing substantial morbidity and loss of mobility. Deterioration in quality of life is severe, with high levels of depression, pain and isolation. Ulcers predominantly affect people over 60 years of age, so that the burden on society is expected to increase with the changing age structure of the population. A major impact on the health services is in community care in which, in the UK, one third of district nursing time is spent dressing leg ulcers. Overall, around 2% of total health expenditure in the UK is spent in the treatment of venous disease, mostly on surgery and community care. This burden in society is unlikely to decrease until much more is known about what steps can be taken to prevent venous disease and impact on the epidemiology.

Key Summary

◆ Around one third of adults with no obvious venous disease have evidence of abnormal valvular incompetence.

◆ Telangiectasia and reticular varices are very common, occurring in around 80% of the adult population.

◆ Trunk varicose veins occur in one quarter to one third of women. Prevalence has been lower in men but may be increasing.

◆ Prevalence of trunk varicose veins increases with age and is probably less common in developed countries.

◆ The occurrence of skin changes, such as hyperpigmentation, eczema and oedema, is related to the severity of varicose veins.

◆ Active venous ulcers occur in about 0.3% of the adult population and 1% have an active or healed ulcer.

◆ The incidence of first deep vein thrombosis (DVT) in the general population is five per 10,000 person years and increases dramatically with age.

◆ Parity and obesity, only in women, are related to the risk of developing trunk varicose veins.

◆ Standing, sitting and bowel habit, especially constipation and straining, may be risk factors for varicose veins, but the evidence is inconclusive.

◆ The risk of venous ulcers is related to severity of varicose veins, ambulatory venous pressure, and previous DVT.

◆ Venous disease, especially venous ulcers, may cause distressing symptoms and impact on quality of life. The burden on hospital and community services is substantial.

References

1. Eklöf B, Rutherford R, Bergan J, Carpentier P, Gloviczki P, Kistner R, Meissner M, Moneta G, Myers K, Padberg F, Perrin M for the American Venous Forum International Ad Hoc Committee for Revision of the CEAP Classification. Revision of the CEAP classification for chronic venous disorders: consensus statement. *J Vasc Surg* 2004; 40: 1248-52.

2. Evans CJ, Fowkes FGR, Ruckley CV, Lee AJ. Prevalence of varicose veins and chronic venous insufficiency in men and women in the general population. *J Epidemiol Comm Health* 1999; 53: 149-53.

3. Schultz-Ehrenburg U, Weindorf N, Matthes U, Hirche H. New epidemiological findings with regard to initial stages of varicose veins (Bochum Study I-III). In: *Phlebologie 92.* Raymond-Martinbeau P, Prescott R, Zummo M, Eds. Paris: John Libbey Eurotext, 1992: 234-36.

4. da Silva A, Widmer LK, Martin H, Mall TH, Glaus L, Schneider M. Varicose veins and chronic venous insufficiency - prevalence and risk factors in 4376 subjects in the Basle Study II. *VASA* 1974; 3: 118-25.

5. Beaglehole R, Prior IAM, Salmond CE, Davidson F. Varicose veins in the South Pacific. *Int J Epid* 1975; 4: 295-9.

6. Langer RD, Criqui MH, Denenberg J, Fronek A. The prevalence of venous disease by gender and ethnicity in a balanced sample of four ethnic groups in southern California. *Phlebology* 2000; 15: 99-105.

7. Brand FN, Dannenberg AL, Abbott RD, *et al.* The epidemiology of varicose veins: the Framingham Study. *Am J Prev Med* 1988; 4: 96-101.

8. Coon WW, Willis PW, Keller JB. Venous thromboembolism and other venous disease in the Tecumseh community health study. *Circulation* 1973; 48: 839-46.

9. Maffei FHA, Magaldi C, Pinho SZ, Lastoria S, Pinho W, Yoshida WB, Rollo HA. Varicose veins and chronic venous insufficiency in Brazil: prevalence among 1755 inhabitants of a country town. *Int J Epid* 1986; 15: 210-7.

10. Callam MJ, Harper DR, Dale JJ, Ruckley CV. Chronic ulcer of the leg: clinical history. *Br Med J* 1987; 294: 1389-91.

11. Nelzen O, Bergquist D, Hallbook T, Lindhagen A. Chronic leg ulcers: an underestimated problem in primary health care among elderly patients. *J Epidemiol Comm Health* 1991; 45: 184-7.

12. Fowkes FJI, Price JF, Fowkes FGR. Incidence of diagnosed deep vein thrombosis in the general population: systematic review. *Eur J Vasc Endovasc Surg* 2003; 25: 1-5.

13. Abramson JH, Hopp C, Epstein LM. The epidemiology of varicose veins - A survey of Western Jerusalem. *J Epidemiol Comm Health* 1981; 35: 213-7.

14. Baker SR, Stacey MC, Jopp-McKay AG, Hoskin SE, Thompson PJ. Epidemiology of chronic venous ulcers. *Br J Surg* 1991; 78: 864-7.

15. Wille-Jørgensen P, Jørgensen T, Andersen M, Kirchaff M. Post-phlebitic syndrome and general surgery: an epidemiological investigation. *Angiology* 1991; 42: 397-403.

16. Simpson A, Roderick P. Varicose veins and venous ulcers. Health care needs assessments. http://radcliffe-oxford.com/vvframe.htm (2003).

Chapter 3

Signs and symptoms of venous disease

Katy AL Darvall MB ChB MRCS (Eng), *Research Fellow*
Rachel C Sam MA MB ChB MRCS (Eng), *Specialist Registrar*
Andrew W Bradbury BSc MD MBA FRCS (Ed) *Professor of Vascular Surgery*
Birmingham University Department of Vascular Surgery
Heart of England NHS Foundation Trust, Birmingham, UK

Introduction

History-taking and clinical examination in patients with venous disease helps the clinician to decide upon further investigations. This information is then used in the context of the patient's symptoms and signs to inform decisions regarding treatment. Importantly, the consultation also enables the clinician to explore the patients' expectations of treatment [1].

Clinical assessment

History-taking

When taking a history from a patient presenting with suspected venous disease, several important questions need to be answered:

◆ What symptoms does the patient have? What are they really concerned about?
◆ Are these symptoms and concerns likely to be due to venous disease? If not, what is the underlying pathology?
◆ Has the patient had any previous treatment for venous disease and, if so, what?
◆ Are there any features in the history suggestive of a previous deep vein thrombosis (DVT)?
◆ What effect are the symptoms having on the patient's health-related quality of life (HRQL) and activities of daily living?
◆ What does the patient hope and expect from treatment?

Patients should be asked about neuromuscular symptoms, such as paraesthesia and weakness, and about any back, hip or knee problems that may be the cause of their symptoms. Osteoarthritis, radicular neuropathy, lymphoedema and arterial insufficiency, the latter usually manifesting as intermittent claudication, are all relatively common conditions that frequently co-exist with venous disease, especially in the older patient age groups [2]. Race and ethnic background may be relevant and should be noted [3].

Features suggestive of a previous DVT include a previous lower limb fracture or immobilisation in a plaster cast, joint replacement, a critical illness or prolonged period of bed rest for any reason, the presence of skin changes of chronic venous insufficiency (varicose eczema, ulceration and lipodermatosclerosis [LDS]) and leg swelling (oedema) [4].

Always ask about medications (including warfarin), smoking and alcohol, and about family history; for example, premature thrombotic and/or recurrent problems may be suggestive of an inherited thrombophilia [5-8].

It is especially important to establish what has prompted the patient to seek medical attention for their venous disease. For example, many patients with asymptomatic and uncomplicated varicose veins (VV) may be simply concerned about their future risk of ulceration or thrombosis; most can be reassured. Others are primarily concerned about the appearance of their legs, while some wish to have physical symptoms such as aching and itching relieved. Failure to understand, and therefore meet, the patient's expectations is an important cause of dissatisfaction, complaint and even medico-legal action [9-11]. Even in the best of hands, venous interventions may be associated with complications and these risks are only worth taking if the intervention is likely to result in patient-reported benefits [12-14].

Clinical examination

As in the history-taking, when undertaking the examination do not be tempted to focus in straight away on the manifestations of venous disease (e.g. VV or ulceration). First, consider the patient as a whole and then examine the legs in general. Always examine both legs, even if the patient is only complaining of unilateral symptoms [15]. While so doing, ask yourself the following important questions:

◆ Does this patient have any underlying disease, for example, peripheral arterial disease, diabetes [16], or cardiac/renal failure, which may be relevant to the development, aetiology, investigation and management of their venous disease?
◆ Considering the legs as a whole, is there evidence of other pathology on one or both sides?
◆ In patients with unilateral symptoms, how does the 'bad' leg compare with the 'good' one? Are any differences between the two legs on objective examination consistent with reported differences in symptomatology?
◆ And last, but not least, what is the CEAP classification of the disease?

Patients should always be examined standing, with support if necessary. The position of any VV should be noted, together with any evidence of complications such as skin changes or ulceration. If appropriate, examine for disease of the spine, hips or knees. Note any scars from previous venous, arterial or orthopaedic surgery. Always feel for and note the presence of pulses; if they are impalpable, always measure the ankle-brachial pressure index (ABPI)[17].

Symptoms of venous disease

We believe it is useful to divide the symptoms of venous disease into those that are 'physical' and those that are 'psychological'. Having said that, this is a clinical spectrum, not a precise dichotomy, with a lot of grey between the black and white; and both frequently co-exist in the same patient.

Physical symptoms

A wide range of physical lower limb symptoms have been ascribed to venous disease: most commonly, pain, heaviness, swelling, itching, restlessness and cramps. Symptoms tend to be less troublesome in the mornings, increase over the course of the day, or with prolonged periods of standing and are often ameliorated by the use of support hosiery. The veins themselves have sometimes been described as being tender and this may be a particular feature in premenstrual women or thrombophlebitis. Ankle and foot swelling, which is typically absent in the morning and tends to develop during the day is a common complaint. However, actual swelling, as opposed to a feeling of swelling, is rarely (if ever) a feature of isolated superficial venous reflux. Thus, if oedema is present on examination, deep venous reflux or obstruction and other pathologies such as congestive cardiac failure and lymphoedema should be excluded.

Common clinical experience indicates that there are large numbers of people with significant venous disease who are asymptomatic, while other patients with apparently trivial disease seem to be greatly troubled by their legs. The often poor relationship between the symptoms of venous disease, the signs of venous disease on clinical examination, and the results of investigations such as duplex ultrasound have been noted in a number of clinical and population-based studies [18,19]. When the consultation appears to uncover such a clinical paradox, extra care must be taken to ensure that the patient's needs and expectations are understood and that they are carefully counselled about what can and cannot be achieved by treatment (Figure 1).

Psychological symptoms

These types of symptoms fall into two categories: concerns about cosmesis and concerns about complications, such as DVT and ulceration.

Cosmesis

Many patients who seek medical advice regarding their VV are concerned about the appearance of their legs and related 'lifestyle' issues. These may not be their only, or even their predominant concerns, and they may not even mention them explicitly during the consultation. For example, the presence of venous disease may affect the patient's choice of clothing,

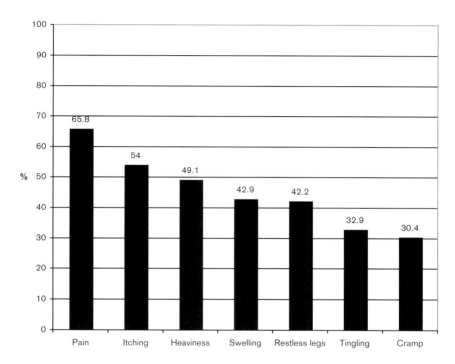

Figure 1 Expectation of relief of physical symptoms: % responding in the affirmative ('quite a bit', 'a lot' or 'an awful lot') to the statement 'I am expecting my VV operation to relieve my lower limb symptoms of...' (based on a cohort of 173 patients undergoing VV surgery).

pursuit of social and leisure activities, their relationships, even their work opportunities (Figure 2). At one end of this clinical spectrum there are those patients with severe disease with whom it is easy to empathise. At the other, there are those patients with unrealistic expectations in whom one suspects an underlying psychological, even psychiatric, problem.

Most patients are aware that they are unlikely to get treatment for VV for cosmetic indications within a publicly-funded health system, such as the UK's National Health Service. Such patients may not mention their cosmetic and 'lifestyle' concerns and may instead invent, or at least inflate,

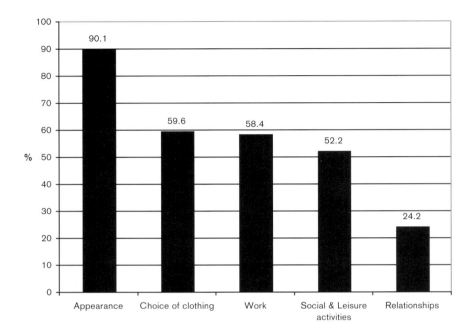

Figure 2 Expectation of lifestyle improvements: % responding in the affirmative to the statement 'I am expecting my varicose vein operation to improve my…' (based on a cohort of 173 patients undergoing VV surgery).

concerns about physical symptoms. It is easy to see how the unwary clinician can find themselves in a doctor-patient relationship where the two parties are working at cross purposes, sometimes with unfortunate consequences. It is difficult to give didactic advice as to how to identify and deal with these patients; to a large extent it only comes through experience. However, the fundamental principles of good history-taking and examination, backed up by careful counselling and meticulous documentation should protect the doctor and the patient from harm.

Complications

Again, common clinical experience allows one to identify those patients who seek medical advice primarily because of concerns that their venous disease will lead to complications, such as DVT and ulceration (Figure 3). The former not infrequently relates to media coverage of 'economy class syndrome' and a forthcoming flight; the latter may arise from experiences with an elderly relative. Again, the patients may or may not explicitly admit to these concerns in the clinic, and such concerns may or may not seem justified. Good communication and history-taking skills employing exploratory and open questions are required to establish understanding, rapport and trust.

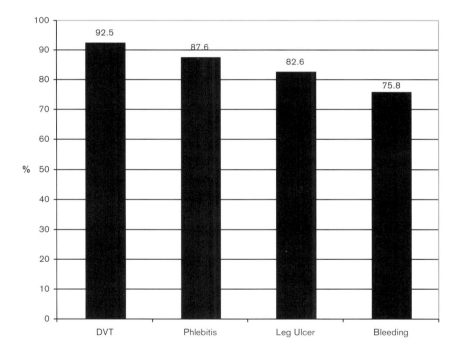

Figure 3 Expectation of reduction in risk of complications: % responding in the affirmative to the statement 'I am expecting my varicose vein operation to reduce my risk of ...' (based on a cohort of 173 patients undergoing VV surgery).

Signs of venous disease

Varicose veins

For descriptive purposes, VV are usually divided into truncal, reticular and hyphenweb varices; the latter are also known as spider veins or telangiectasia.

Trunk varices

These are derived from the great (formerly long) saphenous veins (GSV) and small (formerly short) saphenous veins (SSV) and their first and second order tributaries. They are distinguished from the normally prominent and sometimes dilated superficial veins typically found in the young athletic person by their elongation and tortuosity.

Reticular varices

These are dilated and tortuous subcutaneous veins that do not belong to the main saphenous trunk or its major tributaries. These veins are visible just beneath the skin, sometimes even when normal. These veins typically become dilated in response to back pressure from truncal varices or an incompetent perforating vein. However, in certain patients no obvious source can be found, even on careful clinical and duplex examination.

Hyphenweb varices

These are dilated intradermal venules that can occur in association with trunk or reticular varices or in isolation.

Complications of varicose veins

The complications of varicose veins can be divided into acute (superficial thrombophlebitis and haemorrhage) and chronic (varicose eczema, lipodermatosclerosis, and ulceration).

Superficial thrombophlebitis (SVT)

This commonly involves the GSV and SSV and their major tributaries as a result of an abnormality of one or more of the factors in Virchow's triad (blood flow, vessel wall, blood constituents) leading to thrombosis and secondary inflammation of the vein wall. In the acute phase the patient presents with a painful, tender vein with associated redness and heat. Once the acute stage has 'burned out' the patient is left with hard fibrous cords and lumps and often, if the affected vein is near the skin surface, overlying pigmentation.

Bleeding

This usually follows trauma and the blood loss can be impressive, even life-threatening.

Varicose eczema/stasis dermatitis

This results from the actions of inflammatory mediators released into the skin and subcutaneous tissues as a result of venous hypertension. The skin appears dry, scaly and is often intensely itchy, especially at night. Scratching often leads to bleeding, infection and areas of weeping de-epithelialisation which may form ulcers.

Lipodermatosclerosis (LDS)

This is pigmentation (haemosiderin) and induration of the skin and subcutaneous tissues, as a result of inflammation and the associated increased capillary permeability, which allows the extravasation of red blood cells and protein-rich fluid from the microcirculation.

Chronic venous ulceration

This is normally defined as a break in the skin of the leg present for more than six weeks, that is likely to be due to venous disease. They usually occur in an area of pre-existing LDS as a result of trauma. The majority are in the medial gaiter area with around 20% being laterally placed and 5% circumferential. Venous ulcers are typically shallow, with an irregular margin and a gently sloping edge, and a base of pink granulation tissue, although this may be obscured by yellow-green slough. By contrast, arterial ulcers are usually deep, punched-out lesions with sharp edges and a necrotic base and occur over pressure points. About 1% of leg ulcers are malignant and any longstanding ulcer may undergo malignant change. The clinician should, therefore, have a low threshold for biopsy if there are unusual features, the aetiology is in doubt or the ulcer fails to heal.

Conclusions

Although the advent of duplex ultrasound and, more recently, the availability of affordable, portable machines in the clinic, have transformed the assessment and management of patients with venous disease, the consultation should always start with a careful history and thorough clinical examination. Much can be gleaned from this process, including an understanding of the patient's hopes and expectations of treatment. This can be used to inform investigations and management decisions so that the opportunities for meeting those expectations are maximised, and the risks of disappointment and misunderstanding are minimised [20].

Key Summary

Important features which influence management:

◆ The presence of any other disease process which may account for the patient's symptoms.

◆ The severity and distribution of any varicose veins.

◆ The presence of any complications.

◆ Any previous treatment for venous disease.

◆ Any suggestion of previous DVT.

◆ The patient's hopes and expectations from treatment.

◆ The ability to meet those expectations.

References

1.   Bradbury AW. Modern management of chronic venous insufficiency. *Asian Journal of Surgery* 2003; 26: 129-32.
2.   Ruckley CV, Bradbury AW, Stuart W. Chronic venous ulcer. Causes are often multifactorial and a holistic approach is required. *Br Med J* 1997; 315: 189.
3.   Hobbs SD, Sam R, Rehman A, Marshall T, Wilmink AB, Bradbury AW. The utilisation of superficial venous surgery for chronic venous insufficiency by the U.K. Asian population. *Eur J Vasc Endovasc Surg* 2003; 26: 322-4.
4.   MacKenzie RK, Brown DA, Allan PL, Bradbury AW, Ruckley CV. A comparison of patients who developed venous leg ulceration before and after their 50th birthday. *Eur J Vasc Endovasc Surg* 2003; 26: 176-8.
5.   Bradbury AW, MacKenzie RK, Burns P, Fegan C. Thrombophilia and chronic venous ulceration. *Eur J Vasc Endovasc Surg* 2002; 24: 97-104.

6. Mackenzie RK, Ludlam CA, Ruckley CV, Allan PL, Burns P, Bradbury AW. The prevalence of thrombophilia in patients with chronic venous leg ulceration. *J Vasc Surg* 2002; 35: 718-22.

7. Sam RC, Burns PJ, Hobbs SD, Marshall T, Wilmink AB, Silverman SH. Bradbury AW. The prevalence of hyperhomocysteinemia, methylene tetrahydrofolate reductase C677T mutation, and vitamin B12 and folate deficiency in patients with chronic venous insufficiency. *J Vasc Surg* 2003; 38: 904-8.

8. Sam RC, Wong M, Adam DJ, Fegan C, Silverman SH, Bradbury AW. The association between raised coagulation factor levels and venous thrombo-embolism. *Eur J Vasc Endovasc Surg* 2005; 30: 539-44.

9. Jackson JL, Kroenke KA. The effect of unmet expectations among adults presenting with physical symptoms. *Ann Int Med* 2001; 134: 889-97.

10. Kravitz RL. (2001). Measuring patients' expectations and requests. *Ann Int Med* 2001; 134: 881-8.

11. Campbell WB, France F. Medicolegal claims in vascular surgery. *Ann Roy Coll Surg Eng* 2002; 84: 181-4.

12. Sam RC, Silverman SH, Bradbury AW. Nerve injuries and varicose vein surgery. *Eur J Vasc Endovasc Surg* 2004; 27: 113-20.

13. MacKenzie RK, Lee AJ, Paisley A, Allan PL, Ruckley CV, Bradbury AW. Patient, operative and surgeon factors influencing the effect of superficial venous surgery on disease-specific quality of life. *J Vasc Surg* 2002; 36: 896-902.

14. Hareendran A, Bradbury A, Budd J, Geroulakos G, Hobbs R, Kenkre J, Symonds T. Measuring the impact of venous leg ulcers on quality of life. *J Wound Care* 2005; 14: 53-7.

15. Bradbury AW, Brittenden J, Allan PL, Ruckley CV. Comparison of venous reflux in the affected and non-affected leg in patients with unilateral venous ulceration. *Br J Surg* 1996; 83: 513-5.

16. Cavanagh PR, Lipsky BA, Bradbury AW, Botek G. Treatment for diabetic foot ulcers. *Lancet* 2005; 366: 1725-35.

17. Caruana MF, Bradbury AW, Adam DJ. The validity, reliability, reproducibility and extended utility of ankle to brachial pressure index in current vascular surgical practice. *Eur J Vasc Endovasc Surg* 2005; 29: 443-51.

18. Bradbury AW, Evans CJ, Allan P, Lee AJ, Ruckley CV, Fowkes FGR. What are the symptoms of varicose veins? Edinburgh vein study cross-sectional population survey. *Br Med J* 1999; 318: 353-6.

19. Bradbury AW, Evans CJ, Allan P, Lee AJ, Ruckley CV, Fowkes FGR. The relationship between lower limb symptoms and superficial and deep venous reflux on duplex ultrasonography: The Edinburgh Vein Study. *J Vasc Surg* 2000; 32: 921-31.

20. Sam RC, MacKenzie RK, Paisley AM, Ruckley CV, Bradbury AW. The effect of superficial venous surgery on generic health-related quality of life. *Eur J Vasc Endovasc Surg* 2004; 28: 253-6.

Chapter 4
Investigation of venous disease

Tim A Lees MB ChB FRCS MD

Consultant Vascular Surgeon, Northern Vascular Centre
Freeman Hospital, Newcastle upon Tyne, UK

Introduction

Venous disease occurs most commonly in the legs, probably as a consequence of our erect posture, and this chapter outlines the investigation of venous disease of the lower limb and its complications. The two most common conditions that require investigation on the venous side of the circulation are deep venous thrombosis and varicose veins.

Over the last 15 to 20 years investigation of venous disease has changed, along with many other branches of medicine, to become increasingly non-invasive and more accurate. The aim of investigation is three-fold: firstly, to diagnose the nature of the pathology; secondly, to define the anatomical extent of the problem; and thirdly, to assess the functional consequences. Investigations may be divided into those which provide diagnostic and anatomical information, and those which provide functional information.

Anatomical investigation

Ultrasound scanning

Ultrasound was first used in earnest on the venous side of the circulation in the mid to late 1980s and since then its use has gradually increased, such as it is now frequently the first line, and often the only investigation used in venous disease.

Grey scale B-mode ultrasound provides an anatomical picture of blood vessels and can be used to define the anatomy of the venous circulation, for example, the position of the saphenopopliteal junction, the location of mid-thigh and calf perforating veins, and the presence of connections between the great and small saphenous systems and the superficial and deep venous systems (e.g. Figures 1 to 4). In identifying veins it is rare that B-mode ultrasound will be used in isolation and the addition of Doppler colour flow imaging has greatly enhanced the ability of ultrasound to

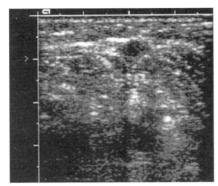

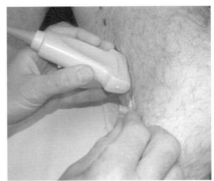

Figure 1 Grey scale B-mode image of small saphenous vein in transverse section, showing as a dark circle within a triangle of fascia.

Figure 2 7.5 MHz Doppler ultrasound probe being used to cannulate the great saphenous vein in the distal thigh.

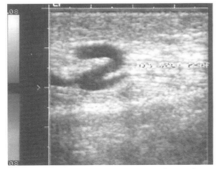

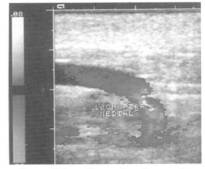

Figure 3 Doppler colour flow images of medial calf perforating veins, showing a tortuous and a straight perforating vein.

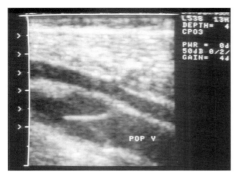

Figure 4 B-mode image of a closed valve in the popliteal vein.

differentiate different types of vessels (see under functional investigation).

Ultrasound tends to perform less well in the pelvis in the identification of iliac vein pathology but even at this site, with modern machines and lower frequency probes, images can usually be obtained.

Ascending venography

Venography used to be the most widely used investigation of venous disease. However, it suffers from the disadvantage of being invasive, it involves the administration of intravenous contrast with a risk of allergy and contrast nephropathy, and as it is used less and less frequently, radiological expertise in its use is decreasing.

Traditional ascending venography is performed by inserting a cannula into a vein on the dorsum of the foot. A tourniquet is then applied at ankle level and contrast is injected. The contrast then passes into the deep system by virtue of the tourniquet occluding the superficial veins at the ankle. X-rays taken of the leg outline the venous system due to the contrast in the veins. Using this method images of the deep system including the iliac veins and the inferior vena cava can be obtained (Figure 5). This method of investigation provides anatomical information and can also be used to diagnose deep venous thrombosis which shows as a filling defect. It also provides some functional information and can be used, for example, to diagnose calf perforating vein incompetence.

Varicography

This involves the direct injection of contrast into a superficial varicosity. This outlines the varicosity including any junctions it may have with other

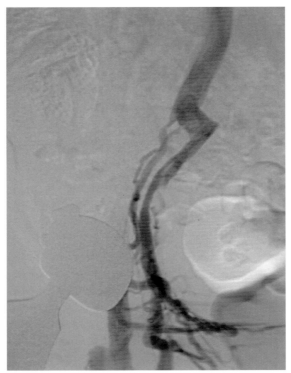

Figure 5 Ascending venogram of the iliac venous system, demonstrating a right external iliac vein occlusion with large collaterals.

superficial veins or the deep venous system. Before ultrasound became widely available it was often used per-operatively to identify the level of the saphenopopliteal junction. Ovarian vein reflux can also be diagnosed by venography of the ovarian veins and if clinically indicated ovarian vein embolisation can be performed. Such patients may present with vulval varicosities and 'pelvic congestion' including pelvic pain, dyspareunia and dysmenorrhoea.

Magnetic resonance imaging (MRI) and computed tomography (CT)

Both of these investigations can provide useful information, particularly on the deep veins of the pelvis, abdomen and chest where access for ultrasound may be difficult. They can provide information on anatomical variations, venous thrombosis, and venous stenosis and occlusion. In the author's practice they have largely superseded venography in the diagnosis of iliac and caval disease and in particular, investigation of the cause of proximal outflow obstruction following deep venous thrombosis.

Both of these investigations can also be used in the diagnosis of pulmonary embolism (see later) and have largely replaced ventilation perfusion scanning for this purpose. They may also identify abdominal, thoracic and pelvic masses causing extrinsic compression of the deep veins.

Functional investigation

Hand-held Doppler examination

The use of hand-held Doppler in the venous clinic is now so commonplace that it may reasonably be considered part of the normal examination of venous disease rather than an investigation. Nevertheless, it is the first-line diagnostic tool used in the diagnosis of venous disease and is therefore included here. The hand-held Doppler uses continuous wave Doppler. The ultrasound beam strikes a moving target (the flowing vein) and is reflected with an altered frequency which can be converted into an audible sound. Hand-held Doppler can therefore be used to listen to sites of suspected venous reflux due to valvular incompetence. The usual sites interrogated are the saphenofemoral and saphenopopliteal junctions. Cephalad flow is induced by either squeezing the calf or asking the patient to dorsiflex the foot and reflux flow, if present, occurs on relaxation. The test can be repeated with manual or tourniquet compression of the superficial veins in order to differentiate superficial and deep venous incompetence.

The disadvantage of hand-held Doppler is that because there is no imaging involved, one cannot be certain as to which vein is being examined and a refluxing vein can easily be missed.

Doppler colour flow imaging (DCFI)

The addition of Doppler to B-mode ultrasound is called duplex scanning. This allows a vessel to be identified and a Doppler trace to be obtained focusing on that individual vessel. This has clear advantages over hand-held continuous wave Doppler in that a specific vein can be identified and then examined for reflux. The Doppler waveform can then be incorporated onto the B-mode image as colour, providing real time images of blood flow within a vessel. Conventionally, flow in one direction is red and flow in the opposite direction is blue, allowing venous reflux to be quickly and easily identified (Figure 6). Reflux flow of greater than one second duration in a vein is usually considered abnormal.

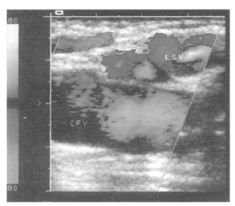

Figure 6 Doppler colour flow image of a recurrent saphenofemoral junction with a tortuous incompetent vein connecting with the common femoral vein.

The patient is usually examined in the erect position in order to maximise the reflux in the examined veins, due to the effect of gravity. A simple scan examining the groin and popliteal fossa can easily be done in five minutes, whereas a detailed scan of the whole lower limb venous tree, particularly in cases of complex pathology, can take up to 30 minutes.

DCFI has the advantage that it is non-invasive and can provide both anatomical and functional information. An argument can be made for performing this investigation on all patients who are being considered for varicose vein surgery, and this is the author's preference. However, it may not be practical to investigate all such patients in this manner due to resource limitations. In this circumstance, straightforward great saphenous vein incompetence can probably be diagnosed using hand-held Doppler alone, but for all other situations, i.e. recurrence, small saphenous reflux, clinical uncertainty, suspected deep venous incompetence, DCFI should be considered.

Descending venography

This is very rarely performed now and will not be discussed in detail here. Essentially, the common femoral vein is cannulated and contrast injected, and a valsalva manoeuvre performed. If the deep venous valves are incompetent, contrast will be seen to flow distally through the incompetent valves.

Functional calf volume measurements

Changes in calf volume indirectly reflect changes in venous filling in the leg. There are various methods which have been used to assess calf volume directly or other parameters which indirectly measure changes in volume. These are called plethysmography, and the main types in current use are photoplethysmography and air plethysmography.

Photoplethysmography [1]

A small probe which emits infrared light is attached to the skin on the medial side of the lower leg. This light penetrates only a short distance into the tissues and is absorbed by the red cells in the subpapillary venous plexus or is reflected back to the probe. The patient performs ten ankle dorsiflexions whilst sitting or standing during which the probe detects a reduction in the content of blood of the cutaneous veins which reflects the changes taking place in the larger veins. A photoplethysmographic venous refilling time can be obtained and this correlates with the ambulatory venous pressure refilling time. The shorter the refilling time the greater the venous reflux in the leg, and so this provides some measurement of the severity of venous disease.

Air plethysmography [2]

There have been several types of air plethysmography developed but the most recent was described by Christopoulos *et al* and is now commercially available. It can be used for the diagnosis of venous reflux and venous outflow obstruction, and the assessment of calf muscle pump function. It consists of an air-filled plastic bag which surrounds the leg from the knee to the ankle. The pressure inside the bag is measured and changes in pressure can be recorded. Following calibration, changes in calf volume can be measured. Various parameters can be recorded. These include:

◆ the venous filling index (ml/sec) which is a measure of the rate of venous reflux in the leg;

◆ the venous outflow fraction which is a measure of venous outflow from the leg;

◆ the ejection fraction which is a measure of how the calf muscle pump ejects blood from the leg; and

◆ the residual volume fraction which is a measure of the volume of the calf following ten tip-toe exercises and therefore reflects the overall combination of venous reflux, venous outflow and calf muscle pump function.

Foot volumetry [3]

The patient stands with both feet in a pair of 'steel boots' and these are filled with water of a known volume. Changes in foot volume can be measured by recording changes in water level in the boots. The patient performs ten knee bends, thereby expelling blood from the foot and calf, and volume expelled and the refilling time can be calculated. This method is not strictly comparable to other methods of functional venous assessment which use tip-toe exercises and ankle dorsiflexions, but nevertheless, is non-invasive and easy to perform, providing a useful assessment of venous function.

Ambulatory venous pressure measurement [4]

This has been the gold standard of functional venous investigation for many years, particularly in the field of venous research. It provides direct measurement of superficial venous pressure at foot level. A vein on the dorsum of the foot is cannulated and connected to a pressure transducer, amplifier and computer to produce a real time computerised graph of pressure against time. The ambulatory venous pressure at the end of ten tip-toe exercises (AVP) can be recorded along with the time taken for the pressure to return to pre-exercise levels (refilling time). More commonly, the 90% refilling time is used (RT90), as this is an easier point on the pressure curve to identify. Patients with venous reflux typically have a higher ambulatory venous pressure and a shorter refilling time.

The author has recently developed a system of continuous ambulatory venous pressure measurement (CAVP), whereby a data monitor can be worn on a belt and connected to a cannula in a foot vein and pressure data over a period of several hours can be recorded. This seems to provide a more physiological assessment of changes in lower limb venous pressure during activity. A typical normal trace of venous pressure against time during different postures and activity is shown in Figure 7.

Normal

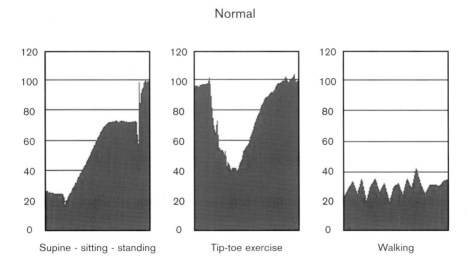

Figure 7 Ambulatory venous pressure trace in a normal individual obtained using a continuous monitoring system, shown for different postures, ten tip-toe exercises, and normal walking.

The investigation of deep vein thrombosis

Deep venous thrombosis is one of the most common clinical venous problems and its sequelae can cause skin changes and ulceration of the leg many years after the initial thrombosis. Prompt diagnosis and treatment to prevent propagation of the thrombus is essential.

Ultrasound has become the mainstay of investigation [5] and has been demonstrated to have a sensitivity and specificity in the region of 97% when compared to venography. However, performing an ultrasound scan on every patient suspected of having a deep venous thrombosis is not practical in terms of resource and, therefore, most centres have developed an algorithm for venous investigation involving clinical risk scoring, screening D-dimer tests and selective ultrasound scanning (see Chapter 12).

D-dimer test

D-dimer is an end product of degradation of fibrin clots which is mediated by plasmin. It can be measured from a blood sample and has been used as a screening test for deep vein thrombosis. Whilst it is not 100% accurate a negative result in the presence of low clinical probability practically rules out deep vein thrombosis [6]. In cases where the clinical probability is intermediate or high it will usually be necessary to proceed to ultrasound scanning.

Compression ultrasound

As for the investigation of venous reflux, ultrasound scanning has become the gold standard for the diagnosis of deep venous thrombosis. Several features of ultrasound in relation to deep venous thrombosis are used and these include:

◆ lack of compressibility of the vein due to the presence of solid thrombus;

◆ loss of spontaneous or normal flow in the vein due to complete or partial occlusion;

◆ loss of phasicity, i.e. normal variation in venous flow with respiration; and

◆ visual thrombus in the vein, although it should be noted that often the grey scale image appears exactly like a patent vein.

Lack of compressibility is the most reliable sign and therefore most commonly used. Figure 8 shows a common femoral vein thrombosis and Figure 9 shows a thrombus in a vein (beneath an artery) causing partial occlusion of the lumen with flow around the thrombus.

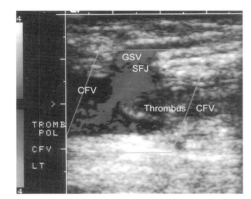

Figure 8 Doppler colour flow image of the saphenofemoral junction with occlusive thrombus in the common femoral vein, extending to the level of the saphenofemoral junction and flow in the great saphenous vein.

Figure 9 Doppler colour flow image of an artery and underlying vein showing a flow-filling defect in the vein due to thrombosis.

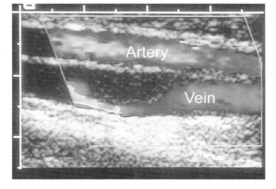

Venography

Venography is an accurate way of diagnosing deep venous thrombosis and used to be the main form of investigation of this condition. However, it has now largely been superseded by ultrasound, CT and MRI.

Magnetic resonance and computed tomography angiography

Both these modalities can be used to examine both peripheral and central veins for the presence of venous thrombosis. In addition, they can be used for pulmonary angiography to diagnose pulmonary embolism [6]. The use of CT in particular has become widespread for this purpose and conventional pulmonary angiography is rarely necessary [7]. A recent review of 13 diagnostic and 11 follow-up studies of CT pulmonary angiography in the diagnosis of pulmonary embolism has demonstrated sensitivities between 53% and 100% and specificities between 79% and 100% [8].

Fibrinogen uptake test

Radiolabelled (^{125} I) fibrinogen has been used to diagnose deep vein thrombosis as this is taken up by a developing thrombus and can be measured by increased radioactivity in the area of the thrombus. Whilst used frequently as a research tool in the past it is now rarely, if ever, used.

Ventilation perfusion scanning

Perfusion lung scanning is performed by the injection of radiolabelled macroaggregates of albumin (usually labelled with $^{99}Tc^m$ technetium), which lodge in the precapillary arterioles. Defects in perfusion of parts of the lung can be detected by a gamma camera. Similarly, inhalation of a technetium-labelled gas (e.g. $^{99}Tc^m$ diethylene triamine-pentacetic acid [DTPA]) can detect areas of reduced ventilation in the lung and therefore areas of ventilation perfusion mismatch can be detected. The limitation of this type of scanning is that there are many other conditions such as emphysema or pneumonia which can produce false positives and therefore CT angiography is a more reliable investigation for the diagnosis of pulmonary embolism.

Conclusions

Technological developments in ultrasound scanning over the last 20 years have led to it now becoming the most widely used investigation of lower limb venous disease. With the range of B-mode scanning, duplex and Doppler colour flow imaging, this non-invasive and harmless investigation can provide anatomical and functional information suitable for most venous diagnostic purposes. If more detailed functional studies are required, plethysmography, foot volumetry and ambulatory venous pressure measurement are still used in specialised centres. Conventional venography, varicography, and isotope studies remain in use but are gradually being replaced by DCFI and other forms of angiography, such as CT and MRI.

Key Summary

◆ Venous investigations can be divided into those that provide information on anatomy and local pathology, such as stenosis and occlusion, and those that assess venous function, such as reflux.

◆ Venography has been the gold standard of venous investigation for many years but this has now been superseded by venous ultrasound which is non-invasive.

◆ Venous ultrasound in the form of Doppler colour flow imaging provides information on venous anatomy, pathology such as deep venous thrombosis, and also venous flow, including reflux, and is therefore in widespread use.

◆ CT angiography, and to a lesser extent MR angiography, have taken over from conventional venography and other investigations in the diagnosis of venous pathology, such as thrombosis, stenosis and occlusion, and the diagnosis of pulmonary embolus.

References

1. Abramowitz HB, Queral LA, Flinn WT, *et al*. The use of photoplethysmography in the assessment of venous insufficiency. A comparison to venous pressure measurements. *Surgery* 1979: 86: 434-41.
2. Christopoulos D, Nicolaides AN. Non-invasive diagnosis and quantitation of popliteal reflux in the swollen and ulcerated leg. *J Cardiovasc Surg* 1988: 29: 535-9.
3. Norgren L. Non-invasive functional investigation of chronic venous insufficiency with special reference to foot volumetry. *Acta Chir Scand Suppl* 1988; 544: 39-43.
4. Nicolaides AN, Zukowski AJ. The value of dynamic venous pressure measurements. *World J Surg* 1986; 10: 919-24.
5. Andrews EJ Jr, Fleischer A. Sonography for deep venous thrombosis: current and future applications. *Ultrasound Q* 2005; 21(4): 213-5.
6. Michiels JJ, Gadissery A, van der Planken M, *et al*. Screening for deep vein thrombosis and pulmonary embolism in outpatients with suspected DVT or PE by the sequential use of clinical score: a sensitive quantitative D-dimer test and non-invasive diagnostic tools. *Semin Vasc Med* 2005; 5(4): 351-64.
7. McRae SJ, Ginsberg JS. Update in the diagnosis of deep vein thrombosis and pulmonary embolism. *Curr Opin Anaesthesiol* 2006; 19(1): 44-51.
8. Hogg K, Brown G, Dunning J, *et al*. Diagnosis of pulmonary embolism with CT pulmonary angiography: a systematic review. *Emerg Med J* 2006; 23(3): 172-8.

Chapter 5
Quality of life and outcome assessment in patients with varicose veins

Alun H Davies MA (Cantab & Oxon) DM (Oxon) FRCS

Reader in Surgery and Consultant Surgeon, Imperial College School of Medicine,
Charing Cross Hospital, London, UK

Nung Rudarakanchana MA MB BChir PhD (Cantab)

House Officer, Charing Cross Hospital, London, UK

Introduction

Varicose veins are one of the most common medical conditions in the Western World with up to 15% of men and 25% of women affected [1]. Each year in the UK, approximately 80,000 varicose vein operations are performed; the independent sector is responsible for about a quarter of these [2]. Varicose vein surgery comprises a significant proportion of the elective surgery workload of vascular surgeons and represents a large percentage of operations on hospital waiting lists. A Scandinavian study found that up to 10% of patients with varicose veins report an inability to work [3]; venous disease accounts for some 0.4% of the total UK invalidity costs in 1992 [4]. In total, management of venous disorders accounts for 1-3% of total healthcare expenditure in this country, translating into over £600 million per year.

What is the relative priority of varicose vein surgery?

Traditionally, varicose vein surgery has been regarded as a low priority procedure and has often been left to be performed by the lowest ranking member of the surgical team. However, there is an emerging body of evidence that well-performed varicose vein surgery has the potential to have a significant impact on lessening the disease burden of patients.

Current National Institute for Clinical Excellence Guidelines state that only patients with complications of varicosities (bleeding, ulcers, superficial thrombophlebitis) or significant symptoms that are having a severe impact on quality of life should be referred on to specialist services [5]. In a survey of members of the Vascular Surgical Society the commonest indications for varicose vein surgery were symptoms (97%) and complications of venous disease (98%). Interestingly, cosmesis was cited as an acceptable indication by 55% of respondents [6]. However, at this time there are no national guidelines stating the specific indications for varicose vein surgery within the National Health Service. Questions regarding patient treatment remain; for example, is surgery appropriate for 'asymptomatic' or uncomplicated, varicose veins? Moreover, the relative priority of varicose vein surgery as compared to other procedures has not been well defined; what priority status should patients on waiting lists for varicose vein surgery have, compared with other common elective procedures? In order to explore these questions, the evidence for varicose vein surgery must be examined and the effectiveness or otherwise of surgical intervention assessed.

Today, surgeons and managers are under increasing pressure to justify the allocation of resources and to prove cost-effectiveness. Robust and specific outcome measures for varicose vein surgery are imperative to rationalising the priority of this procedure within the framework of national health services. This chapter focuses on quality of life and outcome assessment in patients undergoing varicose vein surgery.

Outcome assessment of varicose vein surgery

Due to the heterogeneous population of patients who undergo varicose vein surgery, establishing appropriate endpoints for evaluation is difficult. Indeed, the traditional outcomes of surgical mortality and morbidity would seem to be insufficient to fully illustrate the effects of varicose vein surgery. The outcome of surgical intervention might be assessed in terms of a variety of parameters: subjectively, the individual patient may perceive outcome in terms of improvement in functioning, appearance, and symptoms, often quantified by quality of life and symptom scores; and objectively, the outcome of the procedure may be measured by the rate of recurrence and the prevention of complications. In addition, the adverse sequelae of surgery and the overall cost-effectiveness of the procedure deserve consideration.

Quality of life assessment

Arguably, the most meaningful assessment of an elective intervention is to assess the impact of the intervention on patients' quality of life. Quality of life measures aim to quantify the functional impact of an illness as perceived by the patient. With the increasing burden of chronic diseases, impairment of quality of life is emerging as a relevant symptom, to be considered together with the traditional physical symptoms that the medical profession seeks to alleviate. Both generic and disease-specific measures of perceived health status are used, employing patient questionnaires that are assessed for reliability, validity, responsiveness and practicality. Generic measures are suitable for use across disparate diseases and permit inter-study comparisons and generalisation. Disease-specific health scores target disease-associated effects and are designed to be more sensitive in the detection of specific treatment outcomes.

Generic measures of quality of life

The most widely used generic measure of quality of life is the Short Form 36-item (SF-36) Health Survey. This is well validated in a wide variety of disease states and is able to take into account the impact of comorbidities on health [7]. The questionnaire consists of 36 questions within eight domains, including physical functioning, social functioning, role limitations due to physical or emotional problems, mental health, pain, and health perception. These domains are clustered into two groups: physical health and mental health. Physical health parameters reflect level of functioning whereas mental health components are indicators of well-being. In the SF-36 scoring system, zero represents worst possible health and 100 represents best possible health. Scores may be normalised to the population mean, usually set at 50.

Disease-specific measures of quality of life

The Aberdeen Varicose Veins Questionnaire (AVVQ) is a disease-specific quality of life scoring system developed expressly for patients with varicose veins [8-10]. Designed in 1993, the questionnaire comprises 13 items concerning patient symptoms, including pain, ankle swelling, ulcers and the use of support stockings, and the impact of varicose veins on daily activities, such as interference with social and domestic activities. Consideration is also given to the perceived cosmetic impact of varicosities. Individual questions are weighted to reflect relative contribution to severity by the issues addressed in the question. In the AVVQ scoring system, zero represents no evidence of varicose veins impacting on quality of life and 100 represents the most severe problems associated with varicose veins. The questionnaire has been assessed for reliability, validity, responsiveness and practicality and is proven as a useful measure of quality of life for patients with varicose veins [10].

The VEINES (Venous Insufficiency Epidemiological and Economic Study) quality of life measure is another disease-specific health score that is suitable for assessment of a variety of different clinical presentations of chronic venous disease of the lower limb, including varicose veins and leg ulcers [11]. The VEINES-QOL is available in four different languages (English, French, Italian and French Canadian) and comprises 26 items including ten questions on symptoms (heavy legs, aching legs, swelling, night cramps, heat or burning sensation, restless legs, throbbing, itching and tingling sensation), nine questions on limitations in daily activities, five questions addressing psychological impact, and two questions on changes during the past year and time during the day of highest symptom intensity. Responses are rated on a two to seven-point response scale of intensity, frequency or agreement and higher scores indicate better quality of life. The VEINES-QOL has been rigorously assessed for acceptability, reliability and validity [12].

Symptom assessment

Patients with varicose veins seek medical treatment for a variety of different reasons. Concerns about cosmetic appearance and the possible complications of varicose veins are the most common presentations [13]. A number of patients will present with symptomatic varicosities, most commonly complaining of aching, heaviness and swelling. However, the Edinburgh Vein Study, a large cross-sectional population study, concluded that in patients with demonstrable varices, most lower limb symptoms have a non-venous cause [13]. A minority of patients will present with complications of venous disease, including thrombophlebitis, varicose eczema, lipodermatosclerosis and ulceration. Up to 20% of varicose vein surgery is performed for recurrent varicosities.

More recently, objective scoring systems have been developed for the classification of venous disease severity, enabling validation of studies of different treatment modalities. The CEAP classification (Clinical-Etiology-Anatomy-Physiology) for chronic venous disorders (CEAP 0-6, with higher classes representing more severe disease), recently revised by the American Venous Forum [14], and the Venous Clinical Severity Score (VCSS) [15] are utilised by clinicians to objectively describe the severity of venous disease. A recent study found that physician evaluation of chronic venous disease based on the CEAP classification was significantly correlated with patient-reported quality of life and symptom severity, as measured by the VEINES-QOL questionnaire [16].

Quality of life in patients with varicose veins

Varicose veins impair quality of life

Of the six clinical studies examining generic quality of life scores in patients with varicose veins, as compared to population norms [8, 10, 17-20], four studies demonstrate that patients with varicose veins report significantly worse physical health, but not mental health, than population norms, as reflected by lower SF-36 physical component scores [8, 10, 17, 18]. These results are at odds with the belief, held by some, that varicose veins do not cause significant physical symptoms.

In a large multinational study, Kurz *et al* concluded that the impairment in physical health in patients with varicose veins was associated with concomitant venous disease, such as oedema, skin changes and ulceration, and not the presence of varicose veins *per se* [20]. In this study, the average SF-36 physical component score for women ranged from 47.6 in women with varicose veins alone, to 37.3 in women with varicose veins complicated by ulcer, as compared to the population norm of 50. Interestingly, in women only, the entire spectrum of chronic venous disease affecting the lower limb, including conditions with symptoms or telangiectasia only, was associated with significant compromise in SF-36 mental component scores. However, it should be noted that in this study 65% of the patient cohort were defined as having concomitant disease; given that only 1% of patients with varicose veins are thought to go on to develop ulcers, this sub-population of patients would seem to be over-represented in this study sample. Moreover, patients with symptoms of concomitant disease without varicosities were included, further confounding results.

In order to evaluate the importance of surgical treatment of varicose veins and consider the relative priority of varicose vein surgery, it is relevant to compare the impairment in quality of life in patients with varicose veins to the impairment suffered by patients with other common diseases. Compared to population norms, patients with varicose veins do appear to have impaired quality of life, although their overall SF-36 scores are better than patients with chronic back pain, menorrhagia and suspected peptic ulcer. However, in patients with varicose veins complicated by venous ulceration, SF-36 scores are impaired to a level similar to that of patients with limb limitations (SF-36 scores of 36.5 and 37.7 respectively) and are lower that scores reported by patients with chronic lung disease (42.3), back pain (43.1), or arthritis (43.2) [21].

Outcomes of varicose vein surgery

Quality of life

Varicose vein surgery improves quality of life

Five studies have reported the effects of varicose vein surgery on quality of life measures: two using the SF-36 alone [17, 19], two using the SF-36 in combination with a disease-specific measure [10, 22], and one using the AVVQ alone [23]. All five studies have reported a significant improvement in quality of life in patients following varicose vein surgery. The benefit in terms of SF-36 scores is almost entirely attributable to improvement in physical, rather than mental, component health scores [10, 17, 22]. In the most recent of these studies, Sam *et al* reported significant improvement at two years in the physical functioning and pain component of the SF-36, with respective normalised scores of 42.5 versus 45.3 and 43.8 and 48.9 pre-operatively versus postoperatively [17]. Overall, results from the studies indicate that in fact the benefits of varicose vein surgery, in terms of quality of life, are distinct from the hypothesised improvement in mental health, as a consequence of improved cosmesis. Published reports suggest that the benefits of varicose vein surgery in terms of disease-specific quality of life, as assessed by the AVVQ, are significant and durable out to at least two years postoperatively [22, 23].

MacKenzie *et al* collected and analysed data from 203 patients with chronic venous disease, ranging from symptomatic varicose veins to leg ulcers, who underwent varicose vein surgery. They reported improved AVVQ scores in 86% of patients at six months and 87% of patients at two years following surgical intervention [23]. The group estimated that 40% of the improvement was present at six weeks postoperatively, with an additional 50% up to six months and the remaining benefit cumulating to two years. Data further showed that higher pre-operative AVVQ scores (worse symptoms) correlated with greater improvement in symptoms at two years postoperatively. Moreover, baseline AVVQ scores had a more significant relationship with postoperative AVVQ scores than pre-operative CEAP grade. Thus, this study posited that patients with a high AVVQ score but a low CEAP score may gain more relative benefit, in terms of disease-specific quality of life, from surgical intervention than patients with a low AVVQ score but a high CEAP score.

Symptoms

Early studies aimed at examining the effect of varicose vein surgery focused on patient satisfaction. These studies found that although surgery appeared to improve symptoms, patient satisfaction dropped from 86% at one year to 74% at five years [24]. In one study, only 19% of NHS patients compared with 34% of private healthcare patients were completely satisfied with the outcome of their surgery, whilst 26% of NHS patients and 13% of private patients reported dissatisfaction with their treatment [25]. In a more recent study, complete symptom relief was reported in 63% of men and only 33% of women undergoing varicose vein surgery. However, 88% of men and 75% of women were pleased with the long-term result at a ten-year interval [26]. A proportion of patient dissatisfaction with treatment probably reflects disparity between the patient's and the surgeon's expectations from the procedure, a problem that is amenable to remedy through proper informed consent.

As previously noted, cosmetic concerns are a common presentation of varicose veins; it may be the main incentive for seeking treatment in patients who ostensibly present with other symptoms [24]. However, except for one trial comparing sclerotherapy with surgery, which reported a better cosmetic result in the surgical group at three years [27], there are no objective data as to the effect of varicose vein surgery on cosmesis.

Adverse sequelae

Varicose vein surgery is one of the most common areas for litigation in the UK, accounting for 17% of claims in general surgery. Although regarded by many as a relatively minor surgical procedure, varicose vein surgery does have potential risks of haematoma and wound infection (up to 10%) [28], thrombo-embolism (0.2-0.5% risk of pulmonary embolism) [29], and cutaneous nerve injury (5-7%) [30]. Cases of major vessel or nerve damage have been reported but are very rare. The majority of patients require two to three weeks absence from work following varicose vein surgery [31].

Recurrence

The outcome of surgical intervention most commonly evaluated is the rate of recurrence. However, reported recurrence rates for varicose veins varies widely from 20-80% [32]. The difficulty in assessing surgical treatment by recurrence rates, arises from the fact that there is no agreed definition for recurrence and that recurrence rates vary with length of follow-up and primary method of treatment. Duplex ultrasound demonstrates recurrent reflux in 13-29% of patients at 2-5 years [33-35], whilst clinical recurrence is reported by up to 37% of patients [33, 34]. In the UK, approximately 20% of varicose vein surgery is performed for recurrence; this surgery tends to be more technically demanding and is associated with higher complication rates.

Prevention of complications

The prevalence of venous ulceration in the UK is 0.8-1% [1]. Ulcers may develop in the presence of superficial, deep or perforator reflux. Recent studies have demonstrated that isolated superficial incompetence causes ulcers in 23-53% of cases [36-38] and furthermore, that treatment of varicose veins may improve deep venous haemodynamics [39]. However, the size of varicose veins does not bear a significant relationship to the degree of venous hypertension and the risk of developing ulcers. Up to 40% of patients with leg ulcers and demonstrable superficial reflux do not have visible varicose veins.

It may be hypothesised that prophylactic surgery of patients with asymptomatic or mild varicose veins will prevent skin changes. Once skin changes have occurred surgery may improve the macrocirculation, but has no demonstrable effect on the damaged microcirculation [40]. However, the natural history of varicose veins is largely undocumented and as such it is unknown at what rate patients develop severe venous disease and complications such as skin changes and ulceration. Given the numbers involved (up to 30% of the population), it would seem untenable to advocate surgical intervention without this data.

Whilst it is difficult to resolve the case for prophylactic varicose vein surgery in order to prevent primary venous ulcers, it is possible to assess the effect of surgery on ulcer healing and the risk of recurrent ulceration following healing with compression therapy. One study has demonstrated improved ulcer healing following saphenofemoral junction ligation, but only in patients with isolated saphenous reflux [41]. A second study reported a significant decrease in ulcer recurrence in patients who underwent surgical intervention, as compared to those who declined (9% versus 50%) [42]. In light of this evidence, it may be postulated that varicose vein surgery has a beneficial role in the treatment of venous leg ulcers.

Cost-effectiveness

There are currently no public data on the relative cost-effectiveness of surgery for varicose veins, as compared with other common elective surgical procedures. One randomised controlled trial found that outpatient sclerotherapy was more cost-effective than varicose vein surgery [43]; however, the study was based on information relating to the 1970s and is unlikely to reflect costs in modern practice.

In a study aimed at prioritising waiting lists in terms of expected level of benefit to patients, varicose vein surgery ranked low when considering benefits per resource requirement [44]. However, a separate study recording the clinical condition of 36 patients considered to be at low risk of deterioration of their symptoms whilst waiting a median of 20 months for varicose vein surgery, reported a significant decline in clinical condition and considerable morbidity for patients during the interim [45].

An NHS Health Technology Assessment project was set up in 1998 to examine the cost-effectiveness of the treatment of varicose veins (see www.ncchta.org/projectdata). Due to report later in 2006, the REACTIV (Randomised and Economic Analysis of Conservative and Therapeutic Interventions for Varicose Veins) study aims to assess cost-effectiveness by means of the Markov process decision model, comparing conservative treatment, sclerotherapy and surgery. Patient and social priorities for treatment will be analysed using a 'willingness to pay' technique. The results of this trial are eagerly awaited.

Conclusions

Priority scoring systems have been advocated within the NHS and promote the development of policies that ensure patients on waiting lists are treated on the basis of clinical need [46]. However, national health services operate under all too finite resources and surgeons are under increasing pressure from health authorities to prove treatment cost-effectiveness. Attempts to rationalise the priority of any surgical procedure is required to address both patient need and cost-effectiveness of the treatment.

Varicose veins represent a significant burden of disease, both in terms of the individual patient and the cost to society as a whole. Given non-congruency between lower limb symptoms traditionally considered to be caused by varicose veins and the presence of varicose veins, as exemplified by the Edinburgh Vein Study, it may be argued that a more meaningful 'symptom' to aim to alleviate would be the impairment in quality of life perceived by patients with varicose veins.

Although there is evidence from a number of studies supporting a beneficial role for surgical intervention in patients with varicose veins, there are no randomised controlled trials that include comparisons with non-operative treatment. The placebo effect of surgery cannot therefore be excluded as a significant confounding factor. On balance, however, evidence suggests that varicose vein surgery is a relatively safe operation that is able to substantially relieve symptoms and significantly improve quality of life. Long-term patient satisfaction with the procedure is reasonable, although recurrence rates are appreciable. Whilst the appropriateness of surgical intervention in patients with complications of varicose veins, such as ulcers and thrombophlebitis, is not contested, there is currently no evidence to support the case for prophylactic surgery in the primary prevention of complications of venous disease, such as ulceration. The cost-effectiveness of varicose vein surgery remains to be established.

The majority of varicose vein surgeries are elective procedures, aimed not at decreasing mortality but instead improving morbidity. The significant patient demand for surgical intervention for varicose veins not complicated by ulcers or thrombophlebitis cannot be ignored; the question as to whether it is appropriate for such treatment to be offered by an already struggling public healthcare system is part of a wider issue that needs to be addressed by the medical profession and society as a whole. With a growing proportion of varicose vein surgery taking place in the private sector, it is important that national guidelines are made available and that appropriate regulation of practice is implemented.

Key Summary

◆ Varicose veins significantly impair patients' quality of life.

◆ Surgery for varicose veins significantly improves symptoms and quality of life.

◆ Varicose vein surgery is safe and produces a satisfactory result in the majority of patients.

◆ Recurrence rates are of the order of 25% at ten years but estimates vary.

◆ Surgical intervention is indicated for secondary but not primary prevention of complications of varicose veins, such as ulcers and thrombophlebitis.

◆ Varicose vein surgery may be viewed as a priority elective procedure in terms of patient need.

◆ A randomised controlled trial aimed at defining the cost-effectiveness of varicose vein surgery is due to report later in 2006.

References

1. Callum M. Epidemiology of varicose veins. *Br J Surg* 1994; 81: 167-73.
2. Williams B, McGill J, Rushton L. Private funding of elective hospital treatment in England and Wales, 1997-8: national survey. *Br Med J* 2000; 320: 904-5.
3. Biland L, Widmer LK. Varicose veins and chronic venous insufficiency: medical and socio-economic aspects, Basle study. *Acta Chir Scand* 1988; 544: 9-11.
4. Laing W. Chronic Venous Diseases of the Leg. London: Office of Health Economics, 1992.

5.   Excellence NIoC. Referral advice: a guide to appropriate referral from general practice to specialist services. N0041: London: NICE, 2001.

6.   Lees T, Beard JD, Ridler B, Szymanska T. A survey of the current management of varicose veins by members of the Vascular Surgical Society. *Ann R Coll Surg Engl* 1999; 81: 407-17.

7.   Brazier JE, Harper R, Jones NM, O'Caithin A, Thomas KJ, Userwood T. Validating the SF-36 health survey questionnaire: an outcome measure suitable for routine use within the NHS? *Br Med J* 1992; 305: 160-4.

8.   Garratt AM, Macdonald LM, Ruta DA, Russell IT, Buckingham JK, Krukowski ZH. Towards measurement of outcome for patients with varicose veins. *Qual Health Care* 1993; 2(1): 5-10.

9.   Garratt AM, Ruta DA, Abdalla MI, Russell IT. Responsiveness of the SF-36 and a condition-specific measure of health for patients with varicose veins. *Qual Life Res* 1996; 5(2): 223-34.

10.   Smith JJ, Garratt AM, Guest M, Greenhalgh RM, Davies AH. Evaluating and improving health-related quality of life in patients with varicose veins. *J Vasc Surg* 1999; 30(4): 710-9.

11.   Lamping DL, Abenhaim L, Kurz X, Schroter S, Kahn SR, Group TV. Measuring quality of life and symptoms in chronic venous disorders of the leg: development and psychometric evaluation of the VEINES-QOL/VEINES-SYM questionnaire. *Qual Life Res* 1998; (7): 621-2.

12.   Lamping DL, Schroter S, Kurz X, Kahn SR, Abenhaim L. Evaluation of outcomes in chronic venous disorders of the leg: development of a scientifically rigorous, patient-reported measure of symptoms and quality of life. *J Vasc Surg* 2003; 37(2): 410-9.

13.   Bradbury A, Evans C, Allan P, Lee A, Ruckley CV, Fowkes FG. What are the symptoms of varicose veins? Edinburgh vein study cross-sectional population survey. *Br Med J* 1999; 318(7180): 353-6.

14.   Eklof B, Rutherford RB, Bergan JJ, Carpentier PH, Gloviczki P, Kistner RL, *et al*. Revision of the CEAP classification for chronic venous disorders: consensus statement. *J Vasc Surg* 2004; 40(6): 1248-52.

15.   Rutherford RB, Padberg FT Jr, Comerota AJ, Kistner RL, Meissner MH, Moneta GL. Venous severity scoring: an adjunct to venous outcome assessment. *J Vasc Surg* 2000; (31): 1307-12.

16.   Kahn SR, M'Lan CE, Lamping DL, Kurz X, Berard A, Abenhaim LA. Relationship between clinical classification of chronic venous disease and patient-reported quality of life: results from an international cohort study. *J Vasc Surg* 2004; 39(4): 823-8.

17.   Sam RC, MacKenzie RK, Paisley AM, Ruckley CV, Bradbury AW. The effect of superficial venous surgery on generic health-related quality of life. *Eur J Vasc Endovasc Surg* 2004; 28(3): 253-6.

18.   Kaplan RM, Criqui MH, Denenberg JO, Bergan J, Fronek A. Quality of life in patients with chronic venous disease: San Diego population study. *J Vasc Surg* 2003; 37(5): 1047-53.

19.   Baker DM, Turnbull NB, Pearson JC, Makin GS. How successful is varicose vein surgery? A patient outcome study following varicose vein surgery using the SF-36 Health Assessment Questionnaire. *Eur J Vasc Endovasc Surg* 1995; 9(3): 299-304.

20. Kurz X, Lamping DL, Kahn SR, Baccaglini U, Zuccarelli F, Spreafico G, *et al.* Do varicose veins affect quality of life? Results of an international population-based study. *J Vasc Surg* 2001; 34(4): 641-8.

21. Ware JE Jr, Kosinski MA, Keller SD. SF-36 Physical and Mental Component Summary measures: a user's manual. Boston: The Health Institute, New England Medical Center, 1994.

22. MacKenzie RK, Paisley A, Allan PL, Lee AJ, Ruckley CV, Bradbury AW. The effect of long saphenous vein stripping on quality of life. *J Vasc Surg* 2002; 35(6): 1197-203.

23. Mackenzie RK, Lee AJ, Paisley A, Burns P, Allan PL, Ruckley CV, *et al.* Patient, operative, and surgeon factors that influence the effect of superficial venous surgery on disease-specific quality of life. *J Vasc Surg* 2002; 36(5): 896-902.

24. O'Shaughnessy M, Rahall E, Walsh TN, Given HF. Surgery in the treatment of varicose veins. *Irish Med J* 1989; (82): 54-5.

25. Davies AH, Steffen C, Cosgrove C, Wilkins DC. Varicose vein surgery: patient satisfaction. *J R Coll Surg Edinb* 1995; 40(5): 298-9.

26. Campbell WB, Vijay Kumar A, Collin TW, Allington KL, Michaels JA. The outcome of varicose vein surgery at 10 years: clinical findings, symptoms and patient satisfaction. *Ann R Coll Surg Engl* 2003; 85(1): 52-7.

27. Rutgers PH, Kitslaar PJ. Randomized trial of stripping versus high ligation combined with sclerotherapy in the treatment of the incompetent greater saphenous vein. *Am J Surg* 1994; 168(4): 311-5.

28. Corder AP, Schache DJ, Farquharson SM, Tristram S. Wound infection following high saphenous ligation. A trial comparing two skin closure techniques: subcuticular polyglycolic acid and interrupted monofilament nylon mattress sutures. *J R Coll Surg Edinb* 1991; 36(2): 100-2.

29. Critchley G, Handa A, Maw A, Harvey A, Harvey MR, Corbett CR. Complications of varicose vein surgery. *Ann R Coll Surg Engl* 1997; 79(2): 105-10.

30. Holme JB, Skajaa K, Holme K. Incidence of lesions of the saphenous nerve after partial or complete stripping of the long saphenous vein. *Acta Chir Scand* 1990; 156(2): 145-8.

31. Shamiyeh A, Schrenk P, Huber E, Danis J, Wayand WU. Transilluminated powered phlebectomy: advantages and disadvantages of a new technique. *Dermatol Surg* 2003; 29(6): 616-9.

32. Perrin M. Reconstructive surgery for deep venous reflux: a report on 144 cases. *Cardiovasc Surg* 2000; 8(4): 246-55.

33. Dwerryhouse S, Davies B, Harradine K, Earnshaw JJ. Stripping the long saphenous vein reduces the rate of reoperation for recurrent varicose veins: five-year results of a randomized trial. *J Vasc Surg* 1999; 29(4): 589-92.

34. Jones L, Braithwaite BD, Selwyn D, Cooke S, Earnshaw JJ. Neovascularisation is the principal cause of varicose vein recurrence: results of a randomised trial of stripping the long saphenous vein. *Eur J Vasc Endovasc Surg* 1996; 12(4): 442-5.

35. Turton EP, Scott DJ, Richards SP, Weston MJ, Berridge DC, Kent PJ, *et al.* Duplex-derived evidence of reflux after varicose vein surgery: neoreflux or neovascularisation? *Eur J Vasc Endovasc Surg* 1999; 17(3): 230-3.

36. Labropoulos N, Leon M, Geroulakos G, Volteas N, Chan P, Nicolaides AN. Venous hemodynamic abnormalities in patients with leg ulceration. *Am J Surg* 1995; 169(6): 572-4.

37. Shami SK, Sarin S, Cheatle TR, Scurr JH, Smith PD. Venous ulcers and the superficial venous system. *J Vasc Surg* 1993; 17(3): 487-90.

38. Hoare MC, Nicolaides AN, Miles CR, Shull K, Jury RP, Needham T, *et al.* The role of primary varicose veins in venous ulceration. *Surgery* 1982; 92(3): 450-3.

39. Walsh JC, Bergan JJ, Beeman S, Comer TP. Femoral venous reflux abolished by greater saphenous vein stripping. *Ann Vasc Surg* 1994; 8(6): 566-70.

40. Christopoulos DC, Nicolaides AN, Belcaro G, Kalodiki E. Venous hypertensive microangiopathy in relation to clinical severity and effect of elastic compression. *J Dermatol Surg Oncol* 1991; 17(10): 809-13.

41. Scriven JM, Hartshorne T, Thrush AJ, Bell PR, Naylor AR, London NJ. Role of saphenous vein surgery in the treatment of venous ulceration. *Br J Surg* 1998; 85(6): 781-4.

42. Ghauri AS, Nyamekye I, Grabs AJ, Farndon JR, Whyman MR, Poskitt KR. Influence of a specialised leg ulcer service and venous surgery on the outcome of venous leg ulcers. *Eur J Vasc Endovasc Surg* 1998; 16(3): 238-44.

43. Piachaud D, Weddell JM. The economics of treating varicose veins. *Int J Epidemiol* 1972; 1(3): 287-94.

44. Gudex C, Williams A, Jourdan M, Mason R, Maynard J, O'Flynn R, *et al.* Prioritising waiting lists. *Health Trends* 1990; 22(3): 103-8.

45. Sarin S, Shields DA, Farrah J, Scurr JH, Coleridge-Smith PD. Does venous function deteriorate in patients waiting for varicose vein surgery? *J R Soc Med* 1993; 86(1): 21-3.

46. Edwards RT. Points for pain: waiting list priority scoring systems. *Br Med J* 1999; 318(7181): 412-4.

Chapter 6
Quality of life in patients with venous ulcers

Beverley Sharp MB BS BSc MRCS AKC
Clinical Fellow, Charing Cross Hospital, London, UK
Alun H Davies MA (Cantab & Oxon) DM (Oxon) FRCS
Reader in Surgery and Consultant Surgeon, Imperial College School of Medicine,
Charing Cross Hospital, London, UK

Introduction

In the UK venous ulcers have a prevalence estimated at 1.5-3 per thousand of the population (NHS CRD, 1997) and the economic cost to the NHS is estimated at £300-£600 million a year [1]. Incidence is spread evenly across different socioeconomic groups, but it has been shown that ulcers take longer to heal and recurrence rates are higher in classes IV and V (SIGN, 1998). Prevalence tends to increase with age and therefore the incidence of venous leg ulcers is expected to rise further, as there is a demographic change of increasing numbers of elderly people in the population.

Venous ulcers are a common (80% of all ulcers) [1], chronic and recurring condition. The ulcers involve skin and subcutaneous tissue of the lower limbs occurring mainly at the medial malleolus or gaiter area. They may present with irregular wound edges, ruddy granulation, and a varying degree of yellow fibrotic material in the base. These ulcers tend to be more superficial with infrequent exposure of underlying muscle, tendon, fascia or bone, unless presenting with unrelated pathologies. Exudate levels may vary but are usually moderate to high, and serous in presentation.

Quality of life

The World Health organisation (WHO) has defined health as a state of complete physical, mental and social wellbeing and not merely the absence of disease. WHO defines Quality of Life (QoL) as an individual's perception of their position in life taken in the context of the culture and value systems in which they live and in relation to their goals, expectations, standards and concerns. It is a broad ranging concept affected in a complex way by the person's physical health, psychological state, personal beliefs, social relationships and their relationship to salient features of their environment. It has been alternatively defined by many; for example, van Korlaar describes it as the functional effect of an illness and its consequent therapy upon a patient, as perceived by the patient [2], and Price describes it as the impact of an illness and its treatment on disability and daily living [3].

Determination of the QoL in chronic disease has been assigned increasing scientific attention in recent years for two reasons: firstly, the change in the population age pyramid as previously mentioned; and also the long-term symptom-oriented treatment involved in managing a chronic disease [4]. It is therefore thought that QoL assessment is of great value in highlighting beneficial interventions and management of patients that can then be used to plan further care.

The criteria for an ideal quality of life measure should include equal application to any disease process or outcome, equal application across all levels and degrees of invalidity and proven validity, with a high level of convergence within patient groups when applied across geographic, linguistic and cultural boundaries [5].

Assessment of quality of life

Over recent years there has been ever increasing interest in the QoL of patients with venous ulcers. The assessment of QoL can be divided into generic or specific methods.

Generic methods include the Nottingham Health Profile (NHP) and the Short Form 36-item (SF-36). The NHP was introduced by Hunt, McEwen and McKenna and can be applied to all disease processes [6]. It was designed to provide a brief indication of a patient's perceived emotional social and physical health problems. The SF-36 is a multi-purpose, short-form health survey with only 36 questions that originated in the USA, although this has been anglicised for use in the UK. It yields an 8-scale profile of functional health and wellbeing scores, as well as psychometrically-based physical and mental health summary measures and a preference-based health utility index. It is a generic measure, as opposed to one that targets a specific age, disease, or treatment group. The International Quality of Life Assessment (IQOLA) project was an attempt to translate and adapt the SF-36 questionnaire and validate it in all major languages, thereby making it an international scale of health-related quality of life.

Specific methods include self-report QoL questionnaires that enquire about specific criteria, including the social, physical and psychological conditions of the patient. Authors of these questionnaires include Hyland [7] and Smith [8].

Quality of life of patients with venous ulcers

Not surprisingly, patients with venous ulcers are affected in the physical domain, mostly with regard to pain, physical functioning and mobility. However, it has also been found that they suffer from negative emotional reactions and social isolation [2].

Studies using generic questionnaires have shown that patients with open ulceration (CEAP 6) have a poorer QoL compared to those patients with a healed ulcer (CEAP 5) [9-14]. It has been shown by some that the NHPQ results correlate better with ulcer size, pain, physical mobility, sleep, energy, emotional reaction and social isolation, than the SF-36. Figure 1 shows an example of the difference in QoL as measured between two cohorts of patients with healed and unhealed ulcers.

Examples of specific questionnaires that have been developed include: a self-report questionnaire on QoL, devised by Hyland et al [7], for patients with leg ulcers, focusing on physiological and psychological issues associated with the disease; and the Charing Cross venous ulcer questionnaire, devised by Smith et al [8], addressing social, physiological and psychological issues.

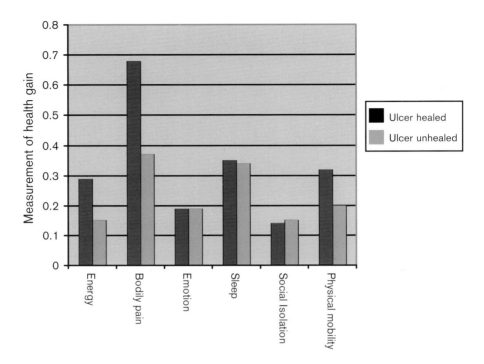

Figure 1 Responsiveness of NHP over 12 weeks treatment in two cohorts of patients with healed and unhealed ulcers. Adapted from data by Franks PJ, Moffatt CJ, 2001 [14].

The advantage of using these specific questionnaires is that it gives a better comparison of specific treatments on the patient's condition.

Conclusions

Sceptics would say that as we know QoL increases with healing and no recurrence of an ulcer, that it is futile to measure the QoL in such patients. The contrary is that the management of patients with venous ulcers is often palliative and hence a treatment offering the patient improved QoL is very beneficial, even if complete ulcer healing is not achieved.

The above has shown that QoL is an important issue in patients with leg ulceration. Furthermore, the use of specific questionnaires can help define optimal treatment plans for patients with venous ulcers.

Key Summary

◆ Venous ulcers cost healthcare systems about 2-4% of their annual expenditure. Venous ulcers are responsible for 80% of all ulcers.

◆ Venous ulcers, as with many chronic diseases, not only inflict physical symptoms on the patient but they have a huge impact on psychological state and social wellbeing which we know equally contribute to a person's health, also referred to as QoL.

◆ Assessment of QoL can be divided into generic or specific methods.

◆ Generic research has shown that patients with open ulceration (CEAP 6) have poorer QoL than those with a healed ulcer (CEAP 5).

References

1. Simon D, Dix F, McCollum C. Management of venous leg ulcers. *Br Med J* 2004; 328: 1358-62.
2. van Korlaar I, Vossen C, Rosendaal F, Cameron L, Bovill E, Kaptein A. Quality of life in venous disease. *Thromb Haemost* 2003; 90(1): 27-35.
3. Price P. Defining and measuring quality of life. *J Wound Care* 1996; 5: 139-40.
4. Metz D. Can the impact of ageing on health care cost be avoided? *J Health Serv Res Policy* 1999; 4: 249-52.
5. Beattie DK, Golledge J, Greenhalgh RM, Davies AH. Quality of life assessment in vascular disease: towards a consensus. *Eur J Vasc Endovasc Surg* 1997; 13: 9-13.

6.   Hunt SM, McEwen J, McKenna SP. Measuring health stats: a new tool for clinicians and epidemiologists. *J Royal Coll Gen Pract* 1985; 35: 185-8.

7.   Hyland ME, Ley A, Thomson B. Quality of life of leg ulcer patients: questionnaire and preliminary findings. *J Wound Care* 1986; 3: 294-8.

8.   Smith JJ, Guest MG, Greenhalgh RM, Davies AH. Measuring the quality of life in patients with venous ulcers. *J Vasc Surg* 2000; 31: 642-9.

9.   Lindholm C, Bjellerup M, Christensen OB, Zederfeldt B. Quality of life in chronic leg ulcer patients. An assessment according to the Nottingham Health Profile. *Acta Derm Venereol* 1993; 73: 440-3.

10. Phillips T, Stanton B, Provan A, Lew R. A study of the impact of leg ulcers on quality of life: financial, social, and psychologic implications. *J Am Acad Dermatol* 1994; 31: 49-53.

11. Franks PJ, Morrell CJ, Culyer AJ, *et al.* Community leg ulcer clinics: effect on quality of life. *Phlebology* 1994; 9: 83-6.

12. Charles H. The impact of leg ulcers on patients' quality of life. *Prof Nurse* 1995; 10: 571-4.

13. Walters SJ, Morrell CJ, Dixon S. Measuring health-related quality of life in patients with venous leg ulcers. *Qual Life Res* 1999; 8: 327-36.

14. Franks PJ, Moffatt CJ. Health-related quality of life in patients with venous ulceration: use of the Nottingham health profile. *Qual Life Res* 2001; 10: 693-700.

Chapter 7
Primary varicose veins: minimising complications, complaint and litigation

Linda de Cossart ChM FRCS

Consultant Vascular and General Surgeon

Countess of Chester NHS Foundation Trust, Chester, UK

Introduction

Performing safe surgery, minimising complications, complaint and litigation requires more than just doing a technically acceptable operation. Superficial varicose veins of the lower limbs are a worldwide problem. Currently in the UK, operative surgery remains the first line of treatment for primary varicose veins of the great and small systems and accounts for about 60,000 operations each year. Vascular specialists have a professional responsibility to do what is best for each individual patient. This can only be achieved by deliberation on a specific patient case [1]. The expectations of surgeon and patient must be established at the start of the case, as in the past, failure to do so has resulted in complications, complaint and sometimes litigation [2].

This chapter is in two parts. The first part emphasises the importance of getting it right before patients get to the operating theatre and provides ideas on how surgeons unpacking their tacit knowledge and understanding might support this. It provides for learners and their teachers a checklist of what they should be thinking about whilst learning venous surgery. The second part describes some technical points arising from the author's own practice.

Getting it right before the operation

Referral to a vascular specialist

Complaint is increasingly an all too familiar part of medical practice. Most complaints (as distinct from litigation) result from a difference in expectation between surgeon and patient. Patients expect their surgeons to treat them with respect, to involve them in deciding between options of treatment for their problem and to provide safe care. When this does not happen they feel driven to complain.

Vocal patients and lay people have encouraged patients to air their complaints and some healthcare organisations have driven the development of very structured complaints procedures and processes [3]. Like complications of operations, complaints can be prevented by careful attention to detail in surgical practice. This will be achieved by surgeons continuing to improve not only their operative expertise but perhaps more importantly, the quality of respect, empathy and imagination they use when engaging with patients. Building on these things throughout a surgical career will not only improve patient satisfaction but will also underpin patient safety.

Litigation (as distinct from complaint) usually ensues when the trust between the patient and their specialist has completely broken down. Campbell *et al* showed that more than half of the claims against surgeons in cases of vascular litigation, followed varicose vein surgery [2]. They concluded that because the cause of many of these claims was failure to advise patients about potential risks and expected benefits, improvements in communication and record keeping would limit future claims. Surgery for varicose veins is rarely a life-saving operation but patients have high expectations of the outcome of such procedures. This must be in the mind of all vascular practitioners as they treat patients with these problems. Mindfulness is the key to reducing litigation.

Preparation for the consultation by the patient and vascular specialist
For the patient, their decision to seek advice about their varicose veins begins with a discussion with their General Practitioner (GP). They may have already talked to others as well as searched the internet. Their GP, recognising the need for an expert opinion, refers the patient to a vascular

surgeon. Therefore, the patient meets the vascular specialist with some preconceived ideas of what they want from the consultation. The vascular surgeon must ensure that they establish a rapport with the patient and elicit from them their expectations. The GP (a professional colleague) will also have an expectation to be informed of the outcome of the consultation. Establishing the expectations of all concerned is an essential first step in a good consultation.

The vascular surgeon will call on more than their knowledge of how to perform the operation at this first meeting. They will need to draw on their knowledge of the range and depth of the subject including the risk-benefit balance for the particular patient, as well as their ability to examine and assess the patient [1]. The vascular specialist's ability to discuss and deliberate these matters with the patient will form the basis for mutual understanding and trust. This will underpin the professional judgement made and avoid unrealistic expectations on each side. Good communication, mutual respect and venous expertise are the cornerstones of safe patient care.

The first outpatient visit

The first outpatient consultation is a critical event and the patient must be given adequate time and consideration. For many patients the first clinic visit may be their only opportunity to discuss their case with an expert. They will remember clearly how they felt at this consultation even if they forget some of the facts offered! The values and personal agenda of the surgeon will be all too obvious to the patient at the consultation, as they establish the history of the patient's complaint, their past medical history (especially considering any previous cardiac, respiratory, thrombo-embolic, anaesthetic, hypertensive, diabetic, limb fracture and injuries, drug allergies), their current drug therapies especially anticoagulant and oestrogen therapy, as well as smoking habits and alcohol consumption. Specific questions of their venous problem should establish venous symptoms and complications (see Table 1). All of these will influence the opinion and the advice given. Most venous operations are now carried out as day cases and follow on from this consultation, but in complex cases or where a patient needs time to consider the options presented at the clinic, a second clinic visit may be necessary. Safe surgery begins long before the operation starts.

The vascular team

The surgeon does not work in isolation but is supported by a clinical team. Those who are delegated tasks by the consultant must understand what these involve and be sure that they are capable of dealing with the responsibilities given to them. This is particularly the case for trainee surgeons who must enter the clinical scenario with a wide range of theoretical knowledge about venous disease and build upon it with clinical expertise learned in practice. A consistent team approach will provide for a stable (and safe) clinical environment. Unfortunately, in the current chaos of British surgical practice this is often missing. Patients are moved between surgeons and even between hospitals in the drive to adhere to targets. This is unsafe practice. Vascular surgeons in the future (those in training and those trained) must strive to create a consistent team approach to ensure a stable (and therefore safer) clinical environment.

Colour flow duplex imaging (CFDI)

Modern duplex imaging has transformed the understanding and management of superficial venous disease. In many centres it is now performed in the outpatient clinic at the first visit. It adds detail to the clinical examination by way of road mapping the anatomy and function of the veins. It is particularly important for surface marking of venous junctions, e.g. the saphenopopliteal junction, as well as identifying variations in anatomy such as two or more great saphenous veins. The CFDI scan must be carried out by vascular surgeons, radiologists, technologists and nurses who understand not only the imaging technique but also the intricacies of venous conditions. In an ideal world all patients should be scanned, but currently limited resources prevent this. As a minimum it is essential to image small saphenous problems and recurrent vein problems, as well as examining the deep veins in patients with a history of deep vein thrombosis (DVT).

Consenting the patient

Obtaining written consent for an operation from the patient is aimed at protecting the surgeon from (in legal terms) assaulting the patient! In the UK there is now a national standard for taking consent for operative procedures which is part of the indemnity process of all NHS Trusts [4]. This is a two-part consent form; the first part is usually filled out and signed by the surgeon (or another competent practitioner) in the clinic following an agreement to proceed with an operation. It must state the operation planned and the complications that may ensue. A copy is given to the patient and one is kept in the notes. An information sheet about varicose veins given to the patient at this time will remind them of the discussion and prepare them to sign the second part of the form prior to surgery. It should be remembered, however, that it is good communication not the consent form that minimises complaint, misunderstanding and accusations of physical assault.

Operating on patients from a common waiting list

In some healthcare systems, varicose veins are often managed on a common waiting list and surgeons therefore find themselves seeing a patient for the first time on the day of surgery. This imposes on them full responsibility for the care of this patient. In so doing they rely heavily on the records and opinions of a colleague as they extract the salient features of the case. Learning to pinpoint the salient features of the case in a rigorous way is essential in minimising complications and complaint by doing the wrong thing! Doing anything less is to act as a technician working on a surgical conveyer belt.

Making practice safer by unpacking a surgeon's tacit knowledge

Working in busy surgical practice does not lend itself to considered reflection on how and what we do. Once a surgical system has been set in place it often remains so for a long time sometimes perpetuating weaknesses that should have been corrected. Young surgeons, who regularly perform venous surgery during their years of training, have rarely been encouraged to take a critical approach to these processes but rather are required to fit in and copy their teacher. Worryingly, this conveyer belt system, that will be an inevitable consequence of the new ways of working in healthcare, will encourage this further. This lack of reflection and critical review is probably what most threatens safe patient care.

The four tables below are set out to offer ideas on what should be in the mind of the practitioner at each step of the patient's journey. Surgeons might use them to reflect on their own practice. For trainees it offers a guide to what they need to learn and how they should think and critically review their practice.

Table 1 What thinking should go on in the mind of the practitioner: in the clinic.

The elements	Your actions	What you should be thinking
Reading the referral letter and meeting the patient	Look up and greet the patient	How does this patient look? Are they fit and well? If they are young and female, is the problem cosmesis or more complex? Are they pregnant? What is the contraceptive choice? What does the patient think of you? What are their expectations?
Simultaneously taking a history and examining the patient	Ask to see the whole limb	Are there signs of venous hypertension? Are the patient's symptoms due to the varicose veins or something else? Is there a history of DVT? Is there a family thrombophilia history? For women, have there ever been problems in pregnancy? Are you giving the impression of caring about the patient's problem?
Doing or ordering the venous CFDI scan	Feel the veins and maybe do a Continuous Wave Doppler (CWD)	Is it clinically a small or great system? Are the foot pulses normal? If you do a scan are you involving the patient in what is going on?

Table 1 *Continued:*

The elements	Your actions	What you should be thinking
Risk-benefit analysis	Provide a risk-benefit analysis for the patient's case	Am I using appropriate statistics and words to express what I mean? Does the patient understand? Have I made a clear distinction between cosmesis and complications of venous disease?
Agreeing a plan	Explain your findings and put them in context to the patient	Are you listening to the patient or merely conveying what you want? Do you think you have made things clear? How do you know this? What senses do you use for this?
Taking consent and giving an information sheet	Fill in the paperwork Give information Ask the patient to say what they understand and record their response	Have you covered all areas with respect to this patient? Do they understand? How do you know they do? Should you record what you think about their understanding?
Closing the consultation	Saying good bye and saying what they may expect next	Ensure that they know what will happen next If you think you have spent too long on this case how can you improve your consultation ability? Should you get someone to comment on your performance?

Venous disease *Simplified*

Table 2 What thinking should go on in the mind of the practitioner: on the day of operation.

The elements	Your actions	What you are/should be thinking (tacit knowledge)
Checking consent	Take it yourself or checking that consent taken by someone else is accurate	Is this the right operation for this patient? Which leg is it? Do they understand the procedure and the likely complications? Does the operation planned match the clinical examination and the results of tests, especially the Doppler ultrasound imaging? (Do not assume the previous clinician was correct, even if more senior than you). Is the consent correct, especially indicating the type and side of operation? If you are a trainee: who is supervising me? Who will assist me?
Talking to the patient	Oral discourse with the patient Do they understand risks/ benefits?	Does the patient know who you are? Does the patient have any last minute questions? Is the patient happy to proceed? Is the patient fit for the operation today?
Checking the notes	Read the notes for yourself	Are the notes (including the letters) present and accurate? If the patient is to have antibiotics (in the case of a leg ulcer) what is their drug allergy status? Be sure that you know what else to give if they are penicillin-sensitive. Has the patient had the department standard anti-DVT prophylaxis? Do they need an extended period of anti-DVT prophylaxis or therapeutic prophylaxis?

Table 2 *Continued:*

The elements	Your actions	What you are/should be thinking (tacit knowledge)
Checking the scan result	See, read and make sure you understand the scan	Has the patient had a scan? Is the scan in the notes? Does it accurately describe the operation and support the procedure for which the patient is listed? If the patient has not had a scan: do they need one? If so, can you get it done now? If not, should the procedure be postponed?
Check prophylactic heparin has been given	Ask the ward staff	Consider any further anticoagulation necessary for any reason specific to this patient
Marking the leg	Ensure that the patient has been standing for at least 30 minutes Mark the leg yourself with a permanent marker pen View the limb from the front and the back Agree with the patient that all the veins they are worried about are marked Mark the point of saphenofemoral reflux in the groin, making sure that it is cosmetically positioned (usually above the knicker line in women) Ensure the saphenopopliteal junction is marked when appropriate	Be sure that you have a clear method of marking and understand the relationship of the marks made to the varicose vein Remember that the pen mark may stain the patient's garments Assess the need for a groin shave and ask one of the staff to be ready to do it when the patient is asleep (or do it yourself)

Table 3 What thinking should go on in the mind of the practitioner: in the theatre. *This table should be read in conjunction with the technical points mentioned later in this chapter, which describe some useful hints on surgical technique.*

The elements	Your actions	What you should be thinking
Communicating with the theatre team	Check with the nursing staff that the operating list is correct for this patient (their name and the procedure) Ensure that the anaesthetist knows the position to place the patient Make sure that you have a first assistant	Is there anything that I should correct right now? Is it safe to continue? Is the patient going to be in the correct position for me to start?
Position the patient on the operating table	Do it yourself or instruct the theatre staff	Is the position comfortable for the patient? Is the position right for me? Could I do this sitting down? Does the patient have any joint problems we should look out for?
Preparing the patient	Hand wash and gown yourself Be ready for the patient as soon as they are pushed into theatre Get an assistant to hold the leg Use an antiseptic preparation (usually alcoholic betadine or chlorhexidine) to swab the lower limb from well above the groin incision to the ankle, ensuring all marked areas are cleaned Place the towels in the manner usually done by the team	View the operation site and note any skin abnormalities Pustules and fungal infection will increase wound infection rates and measures to avoid this should be made Make sure that there are no pools of spirit that may ignite, if diathermy is used. Ensure that the towels are neatly secured and that any movement of the limb necessary is possible

Table 3 *Continued:*

The elements	Your actions	What you should be thinking
Making the first incision	Make an incision about 2 to 2.5cm long above (to avoid tattooing) the mark in the groin Dissect out the veins in the groin defining the saphenofemoral junction	Be sure not to tattoo the patient
Dissecting the saphenofemoral junction (for small saphenous surgery - see later)	Dissect the groin down to the saphenofemoral junction	Think about the anatomy of the veins and be sure that you can identify the branches. Be sure that you know which is the great saphenous vein and which is the femoral vein. Be sure that you have seen the saphenofemoral junction and that all branches are divided
Performing the strip	Pass the stripping device (my preferred choice would be inversion stripping which minimises the size of the track)	How do I get the stripper out of the limb with best cosmetic results? Am I suturing the vein to the stripper to facilitate inversion? What will I do if the vein does not strip? What will I do if the vein breaks and an incomplete vein segment only is removed?
Doing the phlebectomies	Make the skin incision and remove the vein branch using vein hooks	Am I using the most cosmetically pleasing knife to make the incision? Could I make the wound any smaller? How does the wound relate to the vein to be avulsed? Should I modify my marking technique? How can I minimise skin flares at the site of the avulsion wound?

Table 3 *Continued:*

The elements	Your actions	What you should be thinking
Closing the wound	Sew the tissues Put on the wound dressing	Am I doing this in the most appropriate and cosmetically pleasing way? Is the wound dressing convenient for the wound and for the patient? Would something else be more suitable?
Bandaging the leg	Apply the compression dressing	Is the dressing regime I am using appropriate? Is this the most appropriate for the patent? Is there something else that would be better? Have I applied it accurately and well enough to be suitable for the length of time it will be on? What do I know about the patient's opinions of these dressings?
Planning the postoperative care	Record the postoperative care plan in the notes Write to the GP	Have I included all details? Have I written to the GP and included all information for them to know how to advise the patient if called to do so at home?
The operation note	Record the operation note in the patient record	Is this clear and accurate (if hand written, is this easily read and will it be comprehensive and clear when read by someone else at a later date). Does it conform to good operating notes?

Table 4 What thinking should go on in the mind of the practitioner: at the follow-up clinic.

The elements	Your actions	What you should be thinking
The postoperative outpatient review	Greet the patient and take an interest in them and do not be cursory or dismissive Ask about and record any problems they have had Ask how long it took them to get back to normal activity following the surgery Ask them to undress and observe the whole leg, inspecting it fully and if appropriate, touch the areas of concern to the patient Keep accurate and detailed notes Record any disappointments Dictate a letter to the GP and where appropriate copy the patient into the correspondence Plan any follow-up or further procedures, including ultrasound imaging	Observe the patient as they come into the consulting room. What is their demeanour and the body language they exhibit? Do they look happy or not? Be sure to explore your observations, especially if the patient seems unhappy Remember that they are inhibited by doctors and may need to be encouraged to express any unhappiness with the outcome of their surgery. Am I encouraging them to explain; do I look interested in their opinion? Is there anything else that I need to record? Have I given a succinct record to the GP? Is it too long and wordy? Consider any further investigations or interventions necessary

Trainees using this process to review their clinical practice will add insights to their practice and will, I argue, refresh, update and identify things that might be improved. They should use the process with the list of common complications of venous surgery in Table 5. Time must be found for this, as it has the greatest potential to improve patient care (and even surgeon satisfaction).

Table 5 Some common complications of venous surgery.

The complication	A cause	Some solutions
'There are still veins and marks on my leg. The surgeon told me he would give me perfect legs'	Poor communication and the surgeon being unrealistic and probably not understanding the expectations of the patient	Better pre-operative understanding of what the patient wants and being realistic about what can be achieved
'The surgeon did not seem interested and spent very little time with me and I had been waiting for an hour'	Lack of empathy and consideration of the patient's needs by the surgeon	Self-reflection by the surgeon on how the patient sees them
Wound infection	Untreated fungal or other infection in the groin	Treat all groin infections prior to surgery
Skin flares not there before	Stretching of the small avulsion wounds	Warn the patient (different skin types will be more prone), beware of wound stretching when avulsing the vein
Residual veins or new varicosities	Failure to remove the veins or appearance of new veins	Ensure that you agree with the patient what is the likely outcome of surgery. See the patient postoperatively and offer further treatment if appropriate
Tingling and numbness of the skin in the area of surgery	Injury or ischaemia to small skin nerves	Warn the patient. Be vigilant in thinking about the nerves and avoiding them during the operation
Extensive numbness and even other motor injuries	Neuropraxia or neurotmesis, due to direct or indirect injury to the nerves, especially those in the popliteal fossa	Attention to operative technique

Table 5 *Continued:*

The complication	A cause	Some solutions
Postoperative groin haematoma which may need to return to theatre, and other haematomas	Blood collection from the vein strip channel	Compress the leg well Close the GSV track opening in the groin
Deep vein thrombosis	Previous history of DVT or complex case	Explore risks with patient and put them into context. DVT very rare in fit young patients
Recurrence	Poor surgery (unlikely) Unknown reasons Problems when you do not warn the patient	Explain the chances of this
Lymphoedema of the calf	Re-do surgery; lymphoedema already present; unknown	Examine legs properly with this in mind and discuss with patient, especially when doing re-do surgery

Some technical points arising from the author's practice

Great and small saphenous vein surgery is routinely performed under general anaesthetic. The steps in this operation are given in Table 3. In this section, several points are made which the author has found to have improved the safety and cosmesis of the surgery, especially when done by trainees.

Technical points for great saphenous vein (GSV) surgery

Improving cosmesis and safety in accessing the saphenofemoral junction
For over 15 years it has been my practice to mark the position of the groin incision at the same time as marking the varicosities limb for

avulsion. A thrill (elicited by cough or CWD) accurately locates the top of the GSV and the incision line can be planned cosmetically related to this. Female patients find it particularly acceptable to keep it inside the bikini area, which is often not achieved when the incision is made with the patient supine. Marking in this way has also resulted in a shorter incision, as well as giving confidence to inexperienced trainees as to where to make the groin incision.

Positioning of the limb for surgery

The externally rotated and flexed position of the lower limb (as used in arterial surgery) is a good position for access to the saphenofemoral junction, because it opens up the femoral triangle. It is a more comfortable position for the surgeon (in my experience) than the widely abducted limb. Limitations to this may be a stiff hip or knee problem.

Approach to the saphenofemoral junction

Pre-operative marking of the top of the GSV means it is the first large vein visualised in the wound. Placing a clip on it as it appears and lifting it into the wound aids blunt dissection down to the saphenofemoral junction and the GSV branches. Bipolar diathermy to coagulate the branches is safe for the experienced operator but ligation and knot tying is probably best for the inexperienced surgeon.

Reducing tissue trauma and improving cosmesis

Inversion stripping of the GSV using the VITALITEC VITASTRIP significantly reduces tissue trauma by minimising the track in the thigh left by the stripped vein. The thin plastic stripper has an eye at each end for suturing the vein and requires only a 3mm exit incision. (Other equally effective strippers are commercially available).

Cosmesis of the scars at avulsion sites is improved by using an ALCON 2.75mm angled ophthalmic slit knife. The double-edged blade allows a clean incision of between 1-2mm, depending on the size of the vein to be avulsed. The incision must avoid the ink mark to avoid tattooing. Minimum stretching and pulling at the avulsion site reduces the risk of flare formation. The incisions require no dressings other than the wool used for the final compression dressing. Patients appreciate removal of the compression bandage after 24 hours, which allows them to shower. They wear a support stocking for a further three weeks.

Technical points for small saphenous vein (SSV) surgery

Small saphenous vein surgery is a more complex procedure than great saphenous surgery, due to the complexity of the anatomy in the popliteal fossa. The operation is usually performed with the patient under general anaesthetic and in the prone position.

Improving the accuracy of small saphenous vein surgery

The accurate marking of the SSV just before or on the operating table allows the incision to be made right over the saphenopopliteal junction. After longitudinally incising the deep fascia, grasping the vein with an artery clip and lifting it into the wound assists blunt dissection down to the junction.

The use of intra-operative CFDI to identify the saphenopopliteal junction at the beginning and at the end of the procedure has, in our unit, reduced the rate of failure to ligate the junction from 40% to significantly less than 1% [5].

Avoiding nerve injury

The surgeon must be constantly mindful of the position of the sural nerve and the peroneal nerve. Injury to the sural nerve in the line of the main incision may be avoided by ensuring that it is not adherent to the vein and inadvertently clipped. Where retraction on any nerve is necessary it must be released every few minutes in order to avoid neuropraxia. The risk of avulsing the sural nerve is reduced by making very accurate dot marks over veins in the calf and avoiding wide sweeping of the tissues under the skin when hooking out the vein.

Conclusions

Advising and operating on patients with primary varicose veins requires from the vascular specialist not only technical expertise but also sound clinical decision making, which calls upon a wide range of knowledge. This chapter has illustrated how bringing these together might avoid complications, complaint and litigation.

Key Summary

◆ Performing safe surgery, avoiding complications, complaint and litigation requires far more than just doing a technically acceptable operation.

◆ Safe surgery begins long before the operation starts.

◆ Respect, empathy, imagination and good operative technique are necessary qualities for surgeons.

◆ Getting treatment right is more difficult in a target-driven healthcare.

◆ Establishing the expectations of the vascular surgeon and the patient are an essential first step.

◆ A team approach will ensure a stable (and therefore safer) clinical environment.

◆ Improvement in practice should be driven by researching practice and not by the need to address complaints.

◆ Rigorous review of patients seen for the first time on the day of surgery is essential.

◆ Lack of a critical approach by surgeons in reviewing their practice is dangerous.

◆ Surgeons need to explore their tacit thinking especially to help trainees.

◆ Pre-operative marking of the saphenofemoral junction improves both the accuracy and cosmesis of the procedure.

◆ On-table imaging of the saphenopopliteal junction improves the accuracy of the surgery.

References

1. de Cossart L, Fish D. *Cultivating a Thinking Surgeon: new perspectives on clinical teaching, learning and assessment.* tfm publishing Ltd.: Shrewsbury, 2005.
2. Campbell WB, France F, Goodwin HM. Research and Audit Committee of the Vascular Surgical Society of Great Britain and Ireland. Vascular Surgical Society of Great Britain and Ireland, Royal College of Surgeons of England, London, UK. Medicolegal claims in vascular surgery. *Ann R Coll of Surg Eng* 2002; 84(3): 181.
3. http://www.dh.gov.uk/PolicyAndGuidance/OrganisationPolicy/ComplaintsPolicy/fs/en.
4. http://www.dh.gov.uk/PolicyAndGuidance/HealthAndSocialCareTopics/Consent/fs/en.
5. Kumar S, Mitchel G, Rosser S, Edwards PR, de Cossart L, Dimitri SK. Colour flow duplex scanning in short saphenous vein surgery: submitted 2005.

Chapter 8
The management of
recurrent varicose veins

Jonothan J Earnshaw DM FRCS

Consultant Surgeon, Gloucestershire Royal Hospital, Gloucester, UK

Introduction

It is generally believed that re-operative varicose vein surgery has higher complication and recurrence rates than primary surgery. Certainly it can provide a technical challenge; surgery for recurrent small saphenous veins can be one of the most difficult procedures undertaken by a vascular surgeon. Indeed, the benefit of some varicose vein surgery has recently been questioned, on the grounds of poor results after small saphenous surgery [1]. A modern vascular surgeon should question whether surgery is the appropriate treatment for each individual with varicose veins, particularly since new non-surgical treatments such as foam sclerotherapy are becoming available. Varicose vein surgery also remains the focal point for litigation against vascular surgeons, so informed consent is a very central part of management [2].

Why do veins recur?

Many patients and their family doctors believe that recurrence is inevitable after primary varicose vein surgery. Whilst there is evidence that visible recurrent veins are common, symptomatic veins that require re-operation are less common, and can be minimised by appropriate surgery [3]. In most cases there is an obvious reason for recurrent varicose veins, and good management requires an accurate diagnosis. There are four main reasons: incorrect diagnosis, poor surgery, neovascularisation and disease progression.

Incorrect diagnosis

This can happen for example when there is failure to identify saphenopopliteal incompetence (SPI) pre-operatively. If only the great saphenous vein (GSV) is stripped, this is likely to lead to early 'recurrence'. This fact is the basis for the argument that duplex imaging should be done routinely before all varicose vein surgery [4].

Poor surgery

It used to be thought that this was the main cause of recurrent varicose veins, as inexperienced surgeons operated unsupervised. In one surgical series, almost two thirds of recurrences were caused by inadequate groin surgery [5]. Yet, even in contemporary series, with surgery performed by a specialist, a small proportion of patients do not have ideal surgery when checked on postoperative duplex imaging [1, 4]. This appears more common for small saphenous veins (SSV) where failure to disconnect the saphenopopliteal junction (SPJ) occurred in 22% of patients in one series, even when guided by pre-operative duplex marking [1].

Neovascularisation

The commonest reason for failure in GSV surgery is neoreflux that develops at the saphenofemoral junction (SFJ) [6]. Many vascular surgeons believe this is caused by growth of new vessels as a result of the surgery, termed neovascularisation, but others deny this exists and suggest it is simply due to expansion of existing tributaries [7, 8]. Most vascular surgeons agree that groin failure is the commonest reason for recurrent varicose veins and this has spawned a huge amount of research effort into its prevention [9].

Disease progression

New incompetence certainly occurs as time goes by and should not be confused with recurrent varicose veins. In one series, routine duplex imaging six weeks after operation identified new incompetence in 20% of legs [10]. This could be ascribed to altered venous haemodynamics as a result of superficial venous surgery.

Informed consent

Many patients with varicose veins have unrealistic expectations about the possibilities of their treatment. First, they may have symptoms entirely unrelated to varicose veins, such as aching or cramp. A good history may detect bilateralality of symptoms, which should temper the expectation of any improvement following unilateral surgery. In fact, whatever symptoms are reported, approximately 80% will be cured by surgery. Patients often complain of foot and ankle swelling but the effect of varicose vein surgery is very unpredictable on ankle oedema. In western society, there is also an increasing cosmetic expectation which may not be met, and which in some areas may not be funded for treatment by national health agencies.

Before surgery is considered, alternative non-surgical methods should be explored. Sometimes simple reassurance is all that is required. Many patients are frightened about developing a leg ulcer and can simply be reassured, particularly if there is no major truncal venous incompetence. Others fear deep vein thrombosis, often as a potential consequence of flying, yet there is no significant evidence that varicose veins are a risk factor for deep vein thrombosis [11]. Compression stockings may alleviate some of the symptoms of varicose veins, and help prevent skin changes such as varicose eczema. They work best for patients with normal shaped legs who have nimble fingers to enable their easy application. Many patients now use flight socks that they buy from an airport, but it is unlikely these will provide adequate compression. For more difficult shaped legs, the help of a trained nurse with access to stocking aids and made to measure hosiery is an excellent alternative. Many patients prescribed stockings, however, do not wear them!

Sclerotherapy

Standard injection sclerotherapy was popularised in the 1970s by surgeons such as Fegan. It fell out of favour in the decades that followed, because of the high recurrence rates, and occasional complications. New techniques such as duplex-guided foam sclerotherapy are described in Chapter 17. The aim is to use duplex imaging to place foam directly into the vein for occlusion. The problem is that both short and long-term outcome data after foam sclerotherapy are lacking. In expert hands occlusion of major superficial veins can be achieved in 80% to 90% of patients at one week, falling to 70% to 80% at six months. There is huge current enthusiasm for foam sclerotherapy, since it is an outpatient procedure that could replace surgery under a general anaesthetic. It seems most suitable to treat patients that are least likely to benefit from surgery. This includes the elderly, who are at risk from anaesthetic complications, and indeed patients with recurrent varicose veins. In the author's opinion, foam sclerotherapy is likely to supersede surgery for the majority of recurrent varicose veins in the next few years.

Surgery for recurrent great saphenous varicose veins

Presently, re-operation remains the gold standard for patients who require treatment of their recurrent varicose veins. The indications for surgery remain the same as for primary varicose veins. These include complications such as a varicose ulcer, phlebitis or varicose eczema [12]. Patients with symptomatic but uncomplicated varicose veins should be advised using NICE guidelines and may be candidates for surgery after informed consent [13].

The intervention should be guided by appropriate investigation. For most patients this means duplex imaging. Counselling can then include the duplex result, which should at least offer an insight into the likely outcome. For example, it may be appropriate to re-operate on a patient who has an intact SFJ or SPJ, despite previous surgery, whereas the finding of deep venous incompetence in association with superficial varices implies that there may be a poor result, even if the superficial veins are obliterated. Many surgeons believe that the presence of an intact incompetent GSV implies that re-operation with stripping will be worthwhile. Individual decisions will necessarily be based on the results of investigation, but the following approaches may be employed.

Standard redo saphenofemoral disconnection with strip and avulsions

Identification of the SFJ may be difficult, particularly if the first surgeon did a formal flush ligation. Most surgeons therefore employ a lateral approach and first identify the common femoral artery in virgin tissue, then moving medially to the common femoral vein and approaching the SFJ from below [14]. Various incisions can be used. This author prefers re-opening and extending a skin crease incision but others employ a vertical approach, as if for arterial surgery. This avoids transection of lymphatics and may reduce the risk of postoperative seroma, although this is equally achieved by vertical deep dissection through the skin crease incision. A medial approach has also been described but has not become popular [15]. Re-ligation of the SFJ should avoid narrowing the common femoral vein, and is best done using a C-clamp and a running prolene suture. If the GSV is still present, the outcome is often dependent on whether it can be stripped. It may be difficult to find the GSV through the groin incision and it is best to mark the distal GSV pre-operatively so that a stripper can be passed up from below during the surgery.

Reverse GSV stripping alone

Re-do groin surgery has significant potential hazards such as damage to the common femoral vein, and wound complications including seroma, infection and haematoma. It may therefore best be avoided, if possible. In many patients who did not have their GSV stripped at the primary operation, there are multiple small (neovascular) connections to the common femoral vein in the groin. If these are small (say less than 3mm in diameter) a good symptomatic result can be achieved simply by stripping the GSV from below, without re-operating on the SFJ [16]. It is not yet clear whether this will result in a higher recurrence rate long-term.

Barrier technology

The last ten years has witnessed a significant amount of research to try and prevent groin recurrence after varicose vein surgery [9]. In approximately two thirds of patients who had a primary operation by a vascular surgeon, recurrent varicose veins are caused by neoreflux in the groin. Whether these are neovascular veins or existing tributaries, technologies that prevent growth of veins or block their progression in the groin may reduce the risk of recurrence. Several surgeons have employed barriers after primary varicose vein surgery following the pioneering work of Glass [17]. He used a silicone patch, but others have used polytetrafluoroethylene (PTFE) patches or a local pectineus fascial flap [18]. In randomised trials, some of these techniques have reduced early recurrence rates after primary GSV surgery. Both PTFE patches and silicone have been investigated to try to prevent recurrence after redo SFJ ligation, but not in a randomised trial [19, 20]. A silicone patch reduced the rate of neovascularisation in the groin on duplex imaging after five years to 9% from 45% in a previous control cohort [19]. It also reduced the rate of recurrent veins from 58% to 26%. In a study of PTFE patching (Figure 1), the recurrence rate in 81 legs treated with a patch after a median of 19 months was 12%, without any major complications [20]. Randomised trials are awaited.

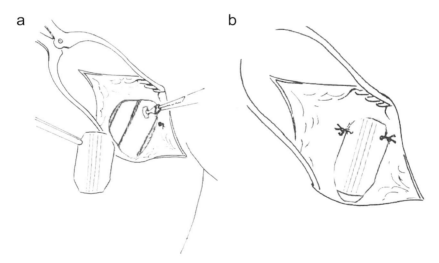

Figure 1 PTFE patch saphenoplasty for recurrent varicose veins. a) The SFJ is religated and the common femoral vein (CFV) exposed over 2-3cm. A 2cm by 3cm PTFE patch is trimmed to fit over the SFJ and exposed CFV. b) The patch is sutured laterally with two 3/0 polyglycolic acid sutures to prevent movement.

New methods of treating varicose veins

There are several new methods available to treat varicose veins. The aim of most novel methods is to try and turn a general anaesthetic inpatient procedure into outpatient surgery under local anaesthesia. Most of the techniques are aimed at primary, rather than recurrent varicose veins. The following section examines their relevance to recurrent vein surgery.

VNUS®

Just like the laser (below), VNUS® is based on thermal destruction of the venous endothelium using radiofrequency ablation. It is a percutaneous technique using endovascular technology and controlled by duplex imaging to create accurate thermal destruction of the endothelium of the GSV. It can be performed using local anaesthetic techniques; this usually involves tumescent local anaesthesia. Several series report high occlusion rates of the GSV, with reduced length of hospital stay and good patient satisfaction [21].

Laser treatment

As for VNUS, the laser technology is aimed at thermal destruction of the endothelium. There were initial problems with venous perforation by the laser wire, but in experienced hands a high rate of venous occlusion can be achieved [22]. There are occasional reports of significant skin burns but these have been overcome by experience and the use of tumescent local anaesthesia. Both VNUS and laser ablation are largely confined to obliteration of long straight veins such as the GSV and SSV. Other tributaries and branches are left for subsequent treatment with sclerotherapy or multiple phlebectomies.

Trivex™

The Trivex machine is a way to harvest superficial varicosities using a device passed through a remote skin incision. The aim is to reduce the number of skin incisions required for phlebectomies and therefore to improve the cosmetic results of varicose vein surgery. The problem is that although the machine is effective and quicker than conventional phlebectomy, it can produce a poor cosmetic result because of the bruising and tissue destruction caused by the device [23]. There are few controlled trials available and the machine has not gained popularity despite several years of availability.

None of these new technologies is specifically indicated for the treatment of recurrent varicose veins. The VNUS and laser techniques may be appropriate in patients with a patent GSV and a small reconnection in the groin. This is the group that may benefit from reverse stripping alone. Trivex may be appropriate in patients who have extensive superficial varicosities but no major vessel incompetence, as an alternative to multiple phlebectomies. Surgical phlebectomies can, however, also be performed as an outpatient using tumescent local anaesthesia.

Surgery for recurrent small saphenous veins

As stated before, this surgery can be extremely difficult; it is also hard to get good results. The same principles of accurate diagnosis, informed pre-operative consent and targeted surgery done by a specialist apply, as for re-operative GSV surgery. Informed consent should particularly include a mention of potential damage to sensory nerves in the popliteal fossa; the majority of surgeons are more likely to warn about this than they are for great saphenous varicose veins [24].

The principal diagnosis is made using duplex imaging, which provides detailed anatomy of the SPJ. In eight out of ten individuals the SPJ is situated near the skin crease in the popliteal fossa, but in 20% it is more than 2cm away, and it can be high in the thigh [25]. This is often the cause of recurrent SSV as there was a failure to ligate the SPJ accurately at the original operation. Recurrence can, however, occur despite apparently adequate surgery done by a specialist with pre-operative duplex marking [1]. When there is abnormal anatomy, pre-operative marking seems sensible, and is done routinely by 47%, and selectively by a further 30% of surgeons [24]. Randomised trials of pre-operative duplex imaging have yet to establish a clear benefit from pre-operative marking.

A technical point is that it is important to mark both the SPJ and the site at which the SSV penetrates the fascia. The SPJ itself may be deep and inaccessible. Most surgeons identify it by exploring the SSV where it penetrates the superficial fascia and then following the SSV down to the SPJ as far as is safe to dissect [24]. This is effective if the distance between the fascial penetration and the SPJ is not excessive. Only a minority of surgeons expose the SPJ anatomically.

Alternative methods of imaging the SPJ include venography and varicography. Although venography has largely been superseded because of the risk of complications, one or two enthusiasts swear by on-table varicography as a means to get an accurate anatomical representation of the SPJ. This has not gained widespread acceptance because of the difficulty of arranging X-rays during the procedure. As many vascular surgeons now operate in endovascular suites, this practice may become more acceptable.

There are many different techniques described for redo SPJ ligation. Most surgeons would use a transverse incision with the patient prone under general anaesthesia. The incision can be extended if necessary and a formal exposure of the SPJ can be achieved. As for primary SSV, there remains controversy as to whether the SSV should be stripped. It is argued that this may increase the risk of cutaneous nerve damage, but in fact many surgeons routinely strip the SSV without evidence of increased sensory deficit. There are no randomised trials to guide the most appropriate management.

Barrier technology has not yet been tested for treatment of SSV and there does not appear to be any advantage of using any new techniques such as VNUS or laser. It has been suggested that simple phlebectomies could be the most appropriate treatment for small saphenous veins to minimise the risk of nerve damage [1], although this means that recurrence is almost inevitable in patients with residual truncal incompetence. There could be a role for Trivex in recurrent small saphenous veins but there are no clinical reports and there remains a significant risk of numbness. With tentative results and outcomes that cannot be guaranteed, there may well be a role for foam sclerotherapy for recurrent SSVs and this promising technology is likely to increase in use as time goes by.

Conclusions

Recurrent varicose veins may be an inevitable consequence of surgical treatment in a proportion of patients. Sometimes it is the fault of the surgeon due to poor technique, but often neovascularisation associated with wound healing, or expansion of existing tributaries due to altered venous haemodynamics initiate recurrence [26]. Prospective studies are few, but suggest that visible recurrent veins occur in a high proportion of patients as the years go by, though a much smaller proportion are symptomatic and require further treatment. Despite the increased risks compared with primary surgery and the fear that re-recurrence is common, surgery remains the gold standard treatment for recurrent varicose veins, in selected patients, and after fully informed consent.

There are currently a number of new less invasive treatments for varicose veins under investigation. The problem is that many of the new techniques may sacrifice durability for a reduction in short-term complications and a speedier convalescence. In itself this may not be a bad thing, but it goes against surgical teaching that flush saphenofemoral disconnection is a vital part of varicose vein treatment. Sceptics may point out that new interventions mainly aim to obliterate major truncal incompetence – perhaps similar results would be obtained if the GSV was simply stripped as primary treatment.

Recurrent veins are fertile ground for venous research, though comparative trials will need to be crafted carefully, and will anyone wait for the long-term results? There are two significant dangers: first, that future interventions for varicose veins will be driven by cost reduction, and second, that they may be driven by industry and advertisement rather than by science and evidence.

Key Summary

◆ Re-operation for recurrent varicose veins is more difficult, less effective and carries higher risks.

◆ Duplex-guided re-operation, and techniques such as routine stripping and possibly barrier technology can reduce the rate of further recurrence.

◆ New methods, such as laser, VNUS and Trivex seem to have little extra to offer over conventional surgery.

◆ It seems foam sclerotherapy is best placed to play a major and increasing role in the management of recurrent varicose veins.

References

1. Rashid HI, Ajeel A, Tyrrell MR. Persistent popliteal reflux following saphenopopliteal disconnection. *Br J Surg* 2002; 89: 748-51.
2. Campbell WB, France F, Goodwin HM. Medicolegal claims in vascular surgery. *Ann R Coll Surg Engl* 2002; 84: 181-4.
3. Winterborn R, Foy C, Earnshaw JJ. Causes of varicose vein recurrence: late results of a randomized controlled trial of stripping the long saphenous vein. *J Vasc Surg* 2004; 40: 634-9.
4. Blomgren L, Johansson G, Bergqvist D. Randomized clinical trial of routine preoperative duplex imaging before varicose vein surgery. *Br J Surg* 2005; 92: 688-94.
5. Stonebridge PA, Chalmers N, Beggs I, Bradbury AW, Ruckley CV. Recurrent varicose veins: a varicographic analysis leading to a new practical classification. *Br J Surg* 1995; 82: 60-2.
6. Jones L, Braithwaite BD, Selwyn D, Cooke S, Earnshaw JJ. Neovascularisation is the principal cause of varicose vein recurrence: results of a randomised trial of stripping the long saphenous vein. *Eur J Vasc Endovasc Surg* 1996; 12: 442-5.
7. van Rij A, Jones GT, Hill GB, Jiang P. Neovascularization and recurrent varicose veins: more histologic and ultrasound evidence. *J Vasc Surg* 2004; 40: 296-302.
8. El Wajeh Y, Giannoukas AD, Gulliford CJ, Suvarna, Chan P. Saphenofemoral venous channels associated with recurrent varicose veins are not neovascular. *Eur J Vasc Endovasc Surg* 2004; 28: 590-4.

Venous disease *Simplified*

9. Fischer R, Chandler JG, De Maeseneer MG, Frings N, Lefebvre-Vilardebo M, Earnshaw JJ, *et al*. The unresolved problem of recurrent saphenofemoral reflux. *J Am Coll Surg* 2002; 195: 80-94.

10. Turton EP, Scott DJ, Richards SP, Weston MJ, Berridge DC, Kent PJ, *et al*. Duplex-derived evidence of reflux after varicose veins surgery: neoreflux or neovascularisation? *Eur J Vasc Endovasc Surg* 1999; 17: 230-3.

11. Campbell WB, Ridler BM. Varicose vein surgery and deep vein thrombosis. *Br J Surg* 1995; 82: 1494-7.

12. Barwell JR, Davies CE, Deacon J, Harvey K, Minor J, Sassano A, *et al*. Comparison of surgery and compression with compression alone in chronic venous ulceration (ESCHAR study): randomised controlled trial. *Lancet* 2004; 363: 1854-9.

13. http://www.nice.org.uk.

14. Gillies TE, Ruckley CV. Surgery for recurrent varicose veins. *Curr Practice in Surg* 1996; 8: 22-7.

15. Greaney MG, Makin GS. Operation for recurrent saphenofemoral incompetence using a medial approach to the saphenofemoral junction. *Br J Surg* 1985; 72: 910-11.

16. Mitton D, Thornton M, Beard JD. Retrograde stripping of recurrent varicose veins. *Eur J Vasc Endovasc Surg* 2001; 22: 90-1.

17. Glass GM. Prevention of recurrent saphenofemoral incompetence after surgery for recurrent varicose veins. *Br J Surg* 1989; 76: 1210.

18. Gibbs PJ, Foy DMA, Darke SG. Reoperation for recurrent saphenofemoral incompetence: a prospective randomised trial using a reflected flap of pectineus fascia. *Eur J Vasc Endovasc Surg* 1999; 18: 494-8.

19. De Maeseneer MG, Vandenbroeck CP, Van Schil. Silicone patch saphenoplasty to prevent repeat recurrence after surgery to treat recurrent saphenofemoral incompetence: long-term follow-up study. *J Vasc Surg* 2004; 40: 98-105.

20. Bhatti TS, Whitman B, Harradine K, Cooke SG, Heather BP, Earnshaw JJ. Causes of re-recurrence after polytetrafluoroethylene patch saphenoplasty for recurrent varicose veins. *Br J Surg* 2000; 87: 1356-60.

21. Lurie F, Creton D, Eklof B, Kabnick LS, Kistner RL, Pichot O, *et al*. Prospective randomised study of endovenous radiofrequency obliteration (Closure) versus ligation and vein stripping (EVOLVeS): two year follow-up. *Eur J Vasc Endovasc Surg* 2005; 29: 67-73.

22. Mundy L, Merlin TL, Fitridge RA, Hiller JE. Systematic review of endovenous laser treatment for varicose veins. *Br J Surg* 2005; 92: 1189-94.

23. Aremu MA, Mahendran B, Butcher W, Khan Z, Colgan MP, Moore DJ, *et al*. Prospective randomized controlled trial: conventional versus powered phlebectomy. *J Vasc Surg* 2004; 39: 88-94.

24. Winterborn RJ, Campbell WB, Heather BP, Earnshaw JJ. The management of short saphenous varicose veins: a survey of members of the Vascular Surgical Society of Great Britain and Ireland. *Eur J Vasc Endovasc Surg* 2004; 28: 400-3.

25. Farrah J, Saharay M, Georgiannos SN, Scurr JH, Coleridge-Smith PD. Variable venous anatomy of the popliteal fossa demonstrated by duplex scanning. *Dermatol Surg* 1998; 24: 901-3.

26. Winterborn RJ, Earnshaw JJ. Crossectomy and great saphenous vein stripping. *J Cardiovasc Surg* 2006; in press.

Chapter 9
New methods of vein ablation

Mark Whiteley MS FRCS (Gen) FRCS (Ed) MB BS
Consultant Vascular Surgeon, The Whiteley Clinic, Guildford, UK

Introduction

The object of therapeutic intervention in superficial venous reflux disease is to stop the reflux of blood from the deep to the superficial system. The commonest site of such reflux is the saphenofemoral junction (SFJ) and so the commonest intervention at present is the high saphenous tie and strip of the great saphenous vein (GSV). This operation [1, 2]:

◆ is usually performed under general anaesthesia;
◆ involves a surgical wound in the groin for the SFJ ligation;
◆ is associated with pain and bruising from the stripping in the thigh; and
◆ involves an exit wound either below the knee or at the ankle.

The early aims of venous ablation techniques were to replace this operation with the following advantages:

◆ to avoid a surgical wound in the groin;
◆ to reduce the pain and bruising in the thigh from stripping;
◆ to enable earlier return to full mobility; and
◆ to give a better cosmetic result.

Once the techniques had become fully developed the aim was also:

◆ to enable treatment under local anaesthetic; and
◆ to enable 'office-based' or 'walk in, walk out' procedures in cases that usually have day-case or 23-hour general anaesthesia.

This chapter will examine the commonest available ablation techniques in more detail and will also examine another potential advantage of the catheter-based thermo-ablation techniques - that of reducing recurrences in the treated vein.

Methods of venous ablation

There are several different techniques of venous ablation that are currently available to interested physicians. As in all areas of a new technology, none of them are perfect and each is continually being modified in terms of the equipment supplied or the operative technique. Each ablation technique has their own intrinsic advantages and disadvantages, and different situations can require different techniques. In our unit, we have found that we regularly need to use combinations of the available techniques to produce the optimal result for our patients.

In order to be able to select the optimal ablation technique, it is worth considering two factors:

◆ the aim of the venous ablation techniques; and
◆ the ablation techniques that are available.

The aim of venous ablation techniques

It is well recognised that open surgery in the groin during the high saphenous tie and strip results in neovascularisation in some cases [3, 4]. We have recently shown that after a high saphenous tie and strip, approximately 20% of people show some regrowth of an incompetent vein within the strip tract within one year. Neither of these findings should really surprise us. It is well documented in wound healing studies that haematoma stimulates endothelial budding from damaged blood vessels within the wound. These buds grow out as solid structures into the area of organising haematoma until they meet other buds. These then join and recanalise making new vessels. Usually called 'wound healing', this is clearly the same process that venous surgeons call 'neovascularisation' [5].

The stimulus for this process to begin is caused by open surgical techniques. These leave both haematoma and damaged blood vessels as part and parcel of the surgery. The body doesn't 'know' that it has had surgery; it has been damaged and so it responds to that insult by trying to heal.

If ablation techniques can avoid the formation of haematoma and can insure that the endothelium is not exposed when the veins are damaged, they should avoid the problems of neovascularisation [6] and strip tract recanalisation [7]. This in turn should reduce the long-term recurrence rates.

In order to ablate a vein permanently, it is preferable (and may be essential) to completely destroy the living cells in the wall, causing transmural death. This will allow the vein wall to fibrose and the body to ingest the dead cells leaving a completely atrophic scar. Destruction of the endothelium alone, or incomplete destruction of the whole wall, allows the possibility of thrombotic occlusion within the venous lumen and a living 'skeleton' of outer media and adventitia. Such a scenario allows recanalisation through the thrombus, using the living venous 'skeleton' as a guide.

The primary aim of venous ablation techniques is therefore to cause transmural death of the vein wall being treated. The avoidance of intra-luminal thrombus will reduce the risks of pain, recanalisation and brown staining of the overlying skin which is due to inflammation and haemosiderin deposition. The avoidance of the vein wall perforation will reduce localised haematoma (bruising) and therefore pain.

In current practice there are two main classes of venous ablation techniques:

◆ catheter thermo-ablation techniques; and
◆ chemical sclerosants.

Catheter-based thermo-ablation techniques

The basic idea of the catheter-based thermo-ablation techniques is to introduce the catheter into the GSV at or below the knee, pass it up the vein under ultrasound guidance to the saphenofemoral junction, and then to switch on an energy source which heats the vein wall and causes transmural ablation. The two methods most commonly used are Radiofrequency Ablation (VNUS Closure®) and EndoVenous Laser (EVL).

Radiofrequency ablation (RFA [VNUS Closure®])

In 1998, VNUS Technologies (California, USA) introduced the VNUS Closure® system for ablating the GSV using a radiofrequency current. There are two different catheters used for smaller or larger veins. When they were first introduced, there was a 5-French Gauge (FG) catheter for the smaller veins and an 8FG catheter for the larger veins. The 5FG catheter has been replaced for several years by a 6FG catheter.

The basic concept of radiofrequency ablation is that a pair of bipolar electrodes is applied firmly to the vein wall and an alternating electrical current is passed between the electrodes at radiofrequencies. The passage of this current between the electrodes is via the vein wall, provided that there is no blood within the lumen and the vein is tightly applied to the catheter. If this is the case, the vein wall becomes heated by 'resistive heating', i.e. heat is generated by the resistance of the cells and proteins to the passage of the alternating current.

Each of the catheters has a thermocouple on one of the electrode blades. This provides feedback of the temperature being generated in the vein wall. By this method, it is possible to accurately heat the vein wall to the target temperature and maintain this heat without overheating the segment. Despite this negative feedback, it is important to remember that the total energy delivered to the wall is a product of the temperature generated and the rate of catheter pull back. If the catheter is moved too quickly, only the inner layers of the vein will be treated; too slow and heat damage to surrounding tissues is possible.

The layout of electrodes in the 6FG catheter is shown in Figure 1. When the catheter is closed it has a blunt end enabling passage up the vein with minimal chance of damage to the endothelium. Once in position the end can be opened and the electrodes exposed. In the 6FG catheter there is one central electrode at the front and a ring of four electrodes behind this. When opened within an exsanguinated vein, the four

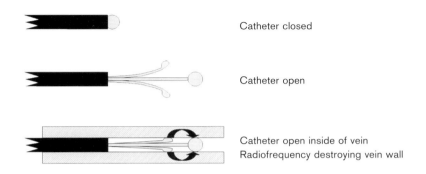

Catheter closed

Catheter open

Catheter open inside of vein
Radiofrequency destroying vein wall

Figure 1 The layout of electrodes in the 6FG catheter.

electrodes come together to act as one ring electrode, with the efficacy current being passed between this and the one central electrode.

The 8FG catheter is obviously bigger and is used for larger diameter veins. Although similar in concept, the 8FG catheter has two rows of electrodes, the central 'ball' being inert in this case and merely there to enable passage of the catheter (Figure 2).

The technique used to close the GSV starts with gaining access to the GSV usually at or below the knee under ultrasound control. The GSV is cannulated with a 14G cannula, a wire passed into the GSV and then using a Seldinger technique, a 6FG or 8FG short sheath is inserted. Once the wire and introducer have been withdrawn, the VNUS catheter can be passed into the vein and advanced to the SFJ. Under ultrasound control, the electrodes are opened at the junction of the inferior epigastric vein. The vein is exsanguinated (the method used depends on anaesthesia, see page 121) and the radiofrequency current is switched on.

Once the temperature has hit the treatment level, the catheter is slowly withdrawn at a prescribed rate, closing the vein as it passes. Initially the recommendation for using radiofrequency ablation was to heat the vein

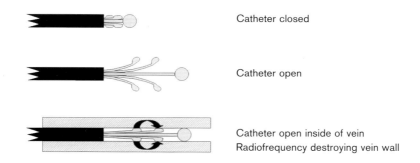

Figure 2 The layout of electrodes in the 8FG catheter.

wall to 85°C. Studies suggested that this gave the optimum protein contraction of the vein wall and our own observations have confirmed complete transmural cell death without loss of vein wall integrity nor perforation. Over the last couple of years there has been a trend to increase the temperature to 90°C which appears to have a similar effect on the vein wall whilst allowing a faster pull back of the catheter and therefore faster treatment.

If blood remains within the lumen of the vein being treated, the heat generated in the wall can cause thrombus which adheres to the electrodes, stopping effective treatment. If this happens, the catheter has to be withdrawn and the electrodes cleaned. The catheter then needs to be replaced and the vein exsanguinated again to ensure adequate treatment. If this is not done, there is the potential for leaving thrombus within the lumen of the vein and an under-treated vein wall. This is a situation that may allow recanalisation in the medium to long term.

Endovenous laser ablation (EVL)

In 1999, Diomed (Cambridge, UK) introduced EndoVenous Laser Treatment (EVLT®) to ablate the GSV using a diode laser. The EVLT®

system uses a wavelength of 810nm and now there are other companies in the marketplace promoting their own EndoVenous Laser systems; there are some variations in equipment or wavelength of the laser used, but the general principle of each is similar.

As with radiofrequency ablation, the GSV is cannulated under ultrasound control. In EVL, an introducer and sheath is passed into the GSV using a Seldinger technique. They are then advanced towards the SFJ. As with radiofrequency ablation, the usual site of stopping is at the junction of the inferior epigastric vein with the GSV. When in position, the wire and introducer are removed and the laser fibre is passed up the sheath. On reaching the end, the sheath is withdrawn leaving the exposed laser fibre in the correct position. An 'aiming beam' is usually used to check the position of the fibre tip (Figure 3).

Treatment begins by switching the laser on. Depending on the wavelength, heat is generated in the blood around the laser tip. With the 810nm systems, steam is produced in the blood around the laser fibre tip and this transmits heat to the vein wall. Longer wavelength systems are being promoted by some as having a direct effect on the proteins on the vein wall, but early laboratory work seems to implicate steam as an intermediary even in these systems.

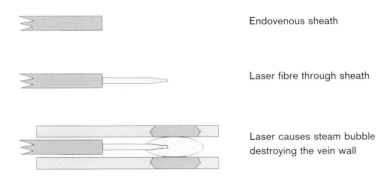

Endovenous sheath

Laser fibre through sheath

Laser causes steam bubble destroying the vein wall

Figure 3 Endovenous laser ablation.

Once switched on, the treatment has commenced and the sheath and laser fibre are withdrawn together - treating the vein as they are pulled down the lumen. Treatment finishes when the sheath and fibre exit the GSV.

Chemical sclerosants

Sclerotherapy has been widely used for decades throughout the world as a treatment for superficial varicose veins. The basic principle of sclerotherapy is to inject a substance into the target vein that destroys the endothelium, hopefully causing a fibrotic healing that keeps the vein closed permanently. However, the injection of such a substance will, by necessity, have an action on any blood cells it comes into contact with, resulting in thrombus within the vein. This can cause pain (thrombophlebitis), brown staining (haemosiderin) and can also result in the recanalisation of the treated section at a later date.

There have been many advances in sclerotherapy techniques over the decades, including the production of the detergent sclerosants, ultrasound guidance to improve placement, exsanguination of the treated vein segment to reduce thrombus formation and making the sclerosants into a micro-foam with gas, which displaces the blood and allows better action of the chemical with the vein wall. Chapter 17 examines sclerotherapy treatments in detail.

However, to put sclerotherapy in context with the catheter-based thermo-ablation techniques, the author's view is as follows. Without doubt these advances have made sclerotherapy a very useful treatment in some areas of venous intervention. However, as even foam sclerotherapy does not cause transmural cell death, the treatment of the large venous trunks with foam sclerotherapy usually leaves living media and adventitia. This 'vein skeleton' is then able to recanalise at any time in the future, leaving the role of sclerotherapy in the treatment of the GSV and small saphenous vein (SSV) in some doubt.

In smaller diameter veins (with thinner walls), sclerotherapy can cause such inflammation that there is transmural cell death. In these situations sclerotherapy is a real alternative to other treatments. Whether it should be used in a particular situation will depend on many factors including, the size and depth of the vein, the alternative treatment methods available, the experience of the operator and the wishes of the patient.

Anaesthesia for venous thermo-ablation

The usual classifications for anaesthesia in medical texts are general, regional or local. With the advent of the minimally invasive thermo-ablation techniques, it may be more useful to classify them into:

◆ Inpatient anaesthesia; and
◆ Outpatient anaesthesia.

Inpatient anaesthesia

The most common inpatient anaesthetic technique is general anaesthesia. As vein surgery is minimally invasive and superficial, there is no requirement for muscle paralysis. Patients can be treated with single-agent infusion anaesthesia (such as Propofol) usually without intubation. The only requirements of general anaesthesia that we have are that the patient is asleep and that Alfentanyl is given. We have discovered that this drug dilates the veins and stops them going into spasm, making percutaneous catheter vein surgery very much easier. Postoperative pain control is achieved by local anaesthetic infiltration of all surgical sites before the patient awakes.

It is also possible to use spinal or epidural anaesthesia, but each of these have potential complications, so that we rarely use them.

There are three advantages in our practice to using general anaesthesia. The first is that we are able to do all the required procedures on one leg in one operative episode. The second is that we can use Alfentanyl for the reasons given above [8]. The problem with using this drug under local anaesthesia is that at the levels needed to cause the desired vasodilatation, the patient stops breathing. This is not a problem under general anaesthesia. The third is that we are able to use a very tight Esmark binding around the leg when using radiofrequency ablation. This is wrapped far tighter than can be tolerated in an awake patient. For radiofrequency ablation to work well, excellent contact between electrodes and vein wall is essential. By using a very thick rubber Esmark bandage wrapped over the whole length of the segment being ablated, we can guarantee exsanguination of the vein at the point of treatment and excellent contact. This is the basis for the excellent closure rates that we have seen in our practice under general anaesthesia with VNUS Closure® (over 99% at 1, 2, 3 and 5 years). These results make this technique the gold standard for GSV treatment in our practice.

In contrast, we would not use EVL under general anaesthesia as the temperatures generated in the vein cause a very steep temperature gradient and the risk to surrounding structures is great. As such, EVL requires tumescence (see below).

Despite the excellent results we obtain using general anaesthesia and VNUS Closure®, there are drawbacks of inpatient anaesthesia. Many people dislike the loss of control and prefer to remain awake during their treatment. The costs of admission, even as a day case, are far more than office-based procedures, even if there needs to be several sessions to produce the same results. These increased costs arise from the higher facility costs charged by hospitals with inpatient facilities, as well as costs for anaesthetic personnel and equipment.

Outpatient anaesthesia

For thermo-ablation techniques, simple local anaesthesia is not sufficient to numb the GSV and to protect the surrounding tissues from thermal damage, particularly with EVL, that can generate intraluminal temperatures in excess of 1000°C. Therefore, the tumescence technique of anaesthesia has been developed.

The GSV sits in a fascial envelope, the saphenous fascia (Figure 4). This is often described as 'The Egyptian Eye'. Once the thermo-ablation device has been passed up the GSV (either VNUS catheter or EVL sheath), ultrasound can be used to identify these structures at all levels in the thigh. Under ultrasound control, a solution of normal saline, local anaesthetic and vasoconstrictor can be injected directly around the GSV but within the saphenous fascia (Figure 5).

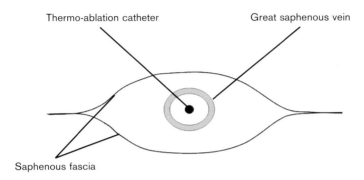

Thermo-ablation catheter

Great saphenous vein

Saphenous fascia

Figure 4 The GSV in a fascial envelope, the saphenous fascia.

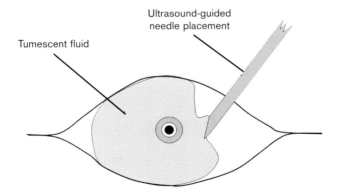

Ultrasound-guided
needle placement

Tumescent fluid

Figure 5 The tumescence technique of anaesthesia.

Infiltration of the saphenous fascia using tumescence this way gives the advantages:

◆ the fluid acts as a 'heat sink' protecting the surrounding tissue from any heat generated in treating the vein;
◆ the local anaesthetic in the solution anaesthetises the vein during treatment;
◆ the pressure of the volume of fluid within the fascial sheath, with the additional effect of the vasoconstrictor in the fluid, constricts the vein around the thermo-ablation device, aiding exsanguination and good vein wall contact.

Our experience with tumescence shows that we would use some 250-400ml to gain an adequate effect in the normal GSV. The two thermo-ablation techniques respond very differently with tumescence.

When using radiofrequency ablation, the pressure produced by the tumescence is not as great as that produced by tight Esmark wrapping under general anaesthesia. Therefore, to close the vein effectively, we usually need manual pressure on the leg in addition to tumescence.

Another area of concern with tumescence and radiofrequency ablation, is the alteration of the physics in the catheter/vein wall action. Radiofrequency heats the vein wall to 85°C or 90°C, depending on chosen value. Although highly effective in a GSV wrapped tightly to the catheter, the tumescent method of anaesthesia changes several factors. Firstly, the vein wall is cooled by the tumescent solution, reducing the effectiveness of the relatively low heats generated on the inner aspect of the vein wall by the radiofrequency catheter. Secondly, the fluid causes some measure of oedema in the vein wall, making it more difficult to get the heat effectively across the vein wall and to cause transmural death.

It is likely to be these factors that result in the late reopening of some GSVs seen in some series using radiofrequency ablation under tumescence. Our experience has shown that an adequately treated GSV will have virtually disappeared on ultrasound by 9-12 months. Those inadequately treated veins that allow a living 'skeleton' of media and adventitia to survive show up by a substantial structure still being visible on ultrasound at 12 months. Such a living 'skeleton' is always capable of allowing recanalisation in the future, often called 'reopening' of the vein.

EVL, with its far higher treatment temperature and its need for haemoglobin as the chromophore to absorb the laser light and turn it to heat, thrives in the environment of tumescent anaesthesia. The high temperatures allow good transfer of heat energy across the vein wall, due to the high temperature gradient helping ensure transmural death. The tumescence then protects other tissues by acting as a heat sink at this point.

Although EVL does perform very well with tumescence, this technique can still have problems. If inadequate power is used (either by setting the power too low or pulling the fibre back too fast) the vein does not undergo transmural death. It either fails to close immediately or re-opens early. On the other hand, too much power causes perforation on the vein wall, allowing blood to escape into the tumescent fluid and cause often extensive bruising. This is both very painful for the patient and might cause either brown staining of the skin or allow neovascularisation to start to be seen as recurrence in the future.

Veins suitable for treatment by venous thermo-ablation

This chapter has concentrated on the treatment of the GSV. These techniques were designed for replacing the high tie and strip and so have been used most commonly to treat this vein. The other veins that can be treated are outlined below.

Second GSV

A second GSV can be found, often as a bifid section. Provided it is within the saphenous fascia, either of the thermo-ablation techniques can be used. If it comes out of the saphenous fascia and becomes more superficial, the skin can be damaged even if tumescence is used to try to push the vein deeper. In these cases we perform avulsion of the vein or, occasionally, foam sclerotherapy if we have already closed the GSV.

Small saphenous vein (SSV)

This is currently one of the areas of great controversy amongst those using thermo-ablation techniques. Due to the difficulty of open saphenopopliteal ligation, endoluminal treatment holds a great appeal. However, the proximity of the lateral popliteal nerve (risking foot drop) and the sural nerve (risking neuralgia or loss of sensation on the lower leg and lateral foot) makes this a vein to be wary of. Current opinion is that the SSV should not be treated by thermo-ablation techniques under general anaesthesia as it is important for the patient to be able to tell the operator that they can feel a shooting pain down the leg. Such symptoms suggest a nerve being heated. Under tumescence, those who perform these procedures usually treat the top 10cm only (reducing the risk of sural nerve damage) and do not let the treatment commence deep in the popliteal fossa. If at any time the patient complains of pain, particularly shooting pain down the leg, the treatment is stopped, the catheter withdrawn 2-3mm and then restarted. If the sensation occurs again, the treatment is again stopped, the catheter withdrawn another 2-3mm and restarted again. This can be repeated until no symptoms are felt.

Although this seems to be the best advice at present, we are waiting for studies to specify the rates of complications to see if such treatment should be common place.

Anterior accessory saphenous vein (or lateral thigh vein) and medial accessory saphenous vein (or medial thigh vein)

When these veins are large, the upper sections are usually straight until they penetrate the superficial fascia. These straight upper sections can be treated by VNUS or EVL as with the GSV. The distal superficial parts are usually varicose and visible and so can be treated by phlebectomy or foam sclerotherapy.

Incompetent perforating veins (IPV)

There is some controversy as to whether IPV need treatment but mounting evidence suggests they are associated with, or cause, recurrences if left untreated at primary varicose vein surgery.

Since 2001 we have been using radiofrequency to close perforators subfascially, a technique we call TRLOP (TRansLuminal Occlusion of Perforators) (Figure 6). Under ultrasound guidance, we cannulate the perforator using a 12G cannula. When in position, a 6FG VNUS Closure catheter is passed into the perforator, opened and the plastic cannula removed. Ultrasound is used to confirm that the electrodes are situated in the IPV, under the deep fascia but outside of the deep vein. When this is achieved, direct pressure is put on the area to ensure good contact and the radiofrequency current switched on. After approximately 50-120 seconds (depending on the morphology of the IPV) the catheter is withdrawn and the IPV checked for patency. Usually the IPV closes first time but it may take up to three attempts to close.

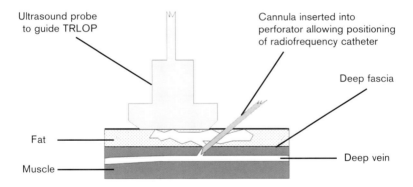

Figure 6 TRansLuminal Occlusion of Perforators.

Giacomini vein

An incompetent Giacomini vein can be closed in its subfascial portion by either VNUS Closure or EVL. However, recent studies have questioned whether an incompetent Giacomini vein ever needs treatment if all other refluxing veins are dealt with. As such, although it is technically possible to treat, the decision as to whether thermo-ablation should be attempted in a Giacomini vein should be made on a case by case basis.

Conclusions

In the excitement of developing these new procedures and techniques, it is important to continually review outcomes. Although at the time of writing this chapter all content is current, things are rapidly changing in this field. There is no doubt that in a year, there will be other products on the market with different profiles and results, and that our unit and others involved in this area, will have produced new techniques or figures that will change our views. This field has changed considerably in the last 12 months, and so it is inconceivable to think that this pace of change won't continue. The following advantages and disadvantages outlined here are only the author's view of the current position.

Advantages

- Reduced pain.
- No groin incision and associated complications.
- Improved return to full mobility and faster return to work.
- Ability to perform in the 'office' as a 'walk in, walk out' treatment.
- Minimal access resulting in very small scars; highly acceptable to patients.
- Probably a reduced recurrence rate as very little neovascularisation has been reported following endoluminal thermo-ablation procedures.
- Popular with patients.

Disadvantages

- A relatively long learning curve, particularly for cases that are not straightforward.
- Requirement for highly skilled vascular technologists / ultrasonographers to diagnose and to guide treatment.
- Requirement for good quality and high resolution ultrasound equipment.
- Training for the doctor, particularly in catheter skills and ultrasound-guided placement of cannulas and catheters.
- Costs, including full diagnostic duplex to plan treatment, increased disposables for treatment, extra ultrasound equipment and staff.

Key Summary

◆ Ultrasound-guided catheter thermo-ablation and sclerotherapy are replacing open surgery for varicose veins.

◆ Thermo-ablation seems to prevent the neovascularisation commonly seen with open surgery.

◆ Minimally invasive techniques are rapidly moving venous surgery into local anaesthetic 'office'-based practices.

◆ Patient advantages include tiny scars, reduced discomfort and minimal 'down-time' from activities.

References

1. Dwerryhouse S, Davies B, Harradine K, Earnshaw JJ. Stripping of the long saphenous vein reduces the rate of re-operation for recurrent varicose veins: five-year results of a randomised trial. *J Vasc Surg* 1999; 29: 589-92.

2. Sarin S, Scurr JH, Coleridge-Smith PD. Stripping of the long saphenous vein in the treatment of primary varicose veins. *Br J Surg* 1994; 81: 1455-8.

3. Glass GM. Neo-vascularisation in the recurrent varices of greater saphenous vein in the groin: phlebography. *Angiology* 1988; 39: 577-82.

4. Jones L, Braithwaite BD, Selwyn D, Cooke S, Earnshaw JJ. Neo-vascularisation is the principal cause of varicose vein recurrence: results of a randomized trial of stripping the long saphenous vein. *Eur J Vasc Endovasc Surg* 1996; 12: 442-5.

5. Glass GM. Neo-vascularisation in the restoration of continuity of the rat femoral vein following surgical interruption. *Phlebology* 1987; 2: 1-6.

6. Kianifard B, Holdstock JM, Whiteley MS. Radiofrequency ablation (VNUS Closure®) does not cause neo-vascularisation at the groin at one year: results of a case controlled study. *Surgeon* 2006; 4(2): 71-4.

7. Varicose veins: endovascular options. Whiteley M. In: *Towards Vascular and Endovascular Consensus*. Roger M Greenhalgh, Ed. London: Biba Publishing 2005: 564-72.

8. Fassiadis N, Scott M, Kianifard B, Holdstock JM, Whiteley MS. Effects of Alfentanil on the diameter of the long saphenous and femoral veins. *Phlebology* 2000; 25: 94.

Chapter 10
Subfascial endoscopic perforator surgery (SEPS)

Monica D Hansrani MD MB BS FRCS, *Specialist Registrar*
Gerard Stansby MChir MB FRCS, *Professor of Vascular Surgery*
Northern Vascular Centre, Freeman Hospital, Newcastle upon Tyne, UK

Introduction

Historically, the calf perforating veins were first described by von Loder in 1803, leading eventually to a description of the 'ankle blow-out syndrome' by Cockett many years later [1]. However, the haemodynamic and clinical relevance of perforator vein insufficiency remains controversial. Indeed, only a small group of patients with chronic venous insufficiency will have isolated perforator incompetence [2]. In patients with advanced disease (CEAP C5, 6), postoperative incompetent perforator veins are a risk factor for recurrence of ulceration [3]. Now that duplex scanning is able to non-invasively assess patients with chronic venous insufficiency, more patients are being discovered who might potentially benefit from medial perforator interruption.

Open perforator surgery

Since the pioneering work of Linton, surgery to divide the medial calf perforating veins has been felt to benefit a proportion of patients with chronic venous insufficiency and leg ulceration [4-7]. However, these operations fell out of favour because of problems with wound healing (in up to 50% of cases in some series), a need for prolonged in-hospital stay and lack of any data showing benefit in the context of a randomised controlled trial with long-term follow-up [8, 9].

Subfascial endoscopic perforator surgery (SEPS)

Albanese in 1965 [10], and Edwards in 1976 [11], described an operation in which a small incision was made in the upper calf and perforators were divided by blunt instruments passed blindly beneath the fascia. Although wound complications were reduced with this operation compared to previous attempts to address perforator disease, it still produced significant complications, including haematoma formation and nerve injury, and it failed to become popular. In 1985, Hauer made a critical advance in this field when he described a new technique where a telescope was introduced into the medial subfascial space through a small incision in the upper calf and then passed down the leg dividing the incompetent calf perforating veins under direct vision. Hauer's initial report of this technique, in the German language [12], was not widely disseminated, however, until the first report in English by Fischer in 1989 [13].

Anatomy for SEPS

Although perforating veins were first mentioned by the Russian anatomist von Loder in 1803, Linton's description in 1938 is more generally known [14]. Cockett first well described the position of the medial calf perforating veins, describing three usual connections between the posterior arch vein and the posterior tibial vena comitantes lying on a perpendicular line originating behind the medial malleolus [15]. Further to this Boyd's perforators connect the same posterior tibial veins to the great saphenous vein (GSV) or the gastrocnemius veins. However, despite numerous pictures and accounts from anatomical texts showing them to be in specific sites, their position and number vary widely between individuals. The majority join the posterior arch vein rather than the GSV and are not reliably disrupted by saphenous stripping. Many also branch or divide just before passing through the fascia and are therefore difficult to divide with small 'stab' incisions. Their inconstancy is the reason duplex marking is recommended prior to a SEPS procedure.

In addition, many of the perforators are 'paratibial' and may require division of the deep fascia to expose them for clipping or coagulation during the SEPS procedure, as they cannot be reached from the medial subfascial approach. This manoeuvre places the posterior tibial vessels at risk and it is essential that the surgeon fully appreciates the anatomy of these vessels with regard to the perforators and the fascial layers. These relationships are not the same at all levels of the calf. Notably, the posterior tibial neurovascular bundle is at greater risk as one approaches the ankle. The anatomy has been well described by Mozes *et al* [16].

Patient selection

There is considerable disagreement regarding patient selection for SEPS. Currently, most of the trials being performed require the patient to have evidence of lipodermatosclerosis, healed ulceration or active ulceration, i.e. class 4, 5 or 6 venous insufficiency on clinical examination, as described by the CEAP classification [9]. The role of SEPS in primary varicose veins is much less clear and the current authors do not recommend its use in uncomplicated varicose veins. In uncomplicated varicose veins, many incompetent calf perforators will become competent after effective control of great or small saphenous incompetence alone. It would seem reasonable therefore to perform a SEPS procedure on CEAP class 4-6 patients who have had the presence of incompetent medial calf perforators demonstrated on duplex scanning, especially if they have failed with conservative treatment or have already had other sites of superficial incompetence ligated [17-20]. The presence of deep venous incompetence is not a contraindication and indeed, patients in this group may derive the greatest benefit. Deep venous obstruction is, however, a contraindication, as the perforating veins will be providing a necessary alternate venous drainage route. Gloviczki *et al* [21] reported a significant increase in non-healing and recurrence of ulceration in deep vein occlusions, whilst others have demonstrated a significantly longer time to ulcer healing in these patients [22].

Technique

It is essential that a full duplex ultrasound assessment of the venous system is carried out. The patient is anaesthetised in the conventional way using either general or spinal anaesthesia. It can easily be performed as a day case if the patient is otherwise fit enough.

After anaesthesia, the leg is prepared and draped in the standard fashion. If saphenofemoral or saphenopopliteal ligation is to be carried out, this is done first. Some surgeons then place a tourniquet on the leg (the most suitable is the Lofqvist roller cuff type tourniquet). This is positioned

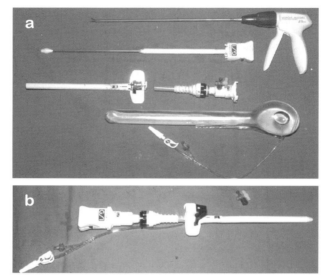

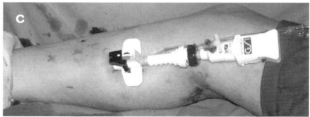

Figure 1 a) Balloon dissection system following separation of the individual components, with the balloon inflated with saline, along with the clip applicator used to clip the perforating veins. b) Balloon subfascial dissection Spacemaker system prior to insertion. c) Spacemaker device following insertion in the subfascial plane. *Courtesy of Tim Lees.*

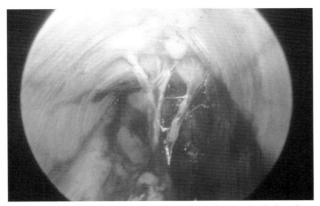

Figure 2 Subfascial view of perforating vein following creation of the subfascial space and insufflation with carbon dioxide. *Courtesy of Tim Lees.*

and then an incision is made over the upper medial calf, away from the area of diseased or ulcerated skin usually two finger-breadths posterior to the tibial margin. The deep fascia is then identified, incised and the telescope introduced under the fascia (Figure 1). The subfascial space is then visualised (Figure 2).

Initially, thoracoscopes or laparoscopes were used, but purpose-made telescopes for the SEPS procedure now exist, using a camera system to display the image on a video as one would for other types of laparoscopic surgery. The telescope can then be passed down the leg in the subfascial space and the perforating veins identified, dissected free and divided. They can be coagulated before division with bipolar diathermy or clipped and then divided. It is also often necessary to divide the fascia close to the tibia with scissors to reach some paratibial perforating veins. In some patients, especially those with severe lipodermatosclerosis, it may be necessary to perform a superficial fasciotomy. This is carried out with a special hook knife that can be introduced down the telescope. This produces more space to work in and may also increase ankle mobility. Other adjunctive techniques include the use of CO_2 insufflation and the use of balloon dissection [23].

Results

Many thousands of these procedures have now been described, mostly in the German literature. After Hauer's original report in 1985, Fischer, in 1989, presented a series of 463 legs treated with this procedure with excellent technical results [13]. Unfortunately, these and other early publications did not detail the types of venous pathology present and the majority of the patients studied did not have ulceration. Jugenheimer and Junginger published a series of 103 legs in 72 patients undergoing the SEPS procedure [24]. As in most other series the majority (94%) had other superficial venous surgery performed at the same time, making it difficult to assess the role of the SEPS procedure alone. There were wound infection problems in 2-9%, neurological lesions in the distribution of the saphenous nerve in 9.7% and haematomas in 5.8%. Patient selection was not well defined and there were no long-term follow-up data.

The first large series to emerge from outside Germany came from Pierik in 1995 [25]. He looked at 40 legs in 38 patients with recurrent or protracted venous ulcers in whom he had identified calf perforator veins, using duplex scanning. He used a mediastinoscope with no tourniquet on the leg to identify and divide the veins. His results were impressive with only one patient developing a recurrent leg ulcer at 3.9 years median follow-up. Of his 40 patients, 31 had associated deep venous incompetence. Only two patients had complications following the operation, one, a wound infection and another, a haematoma, needing drainage. The mean time for the procedure was 21 minutes (range 10-42 minutes). The mean number of perforators divided was 2.4 (range 1-5). More recently the same group has published long-term follow-up on a group of 39 patients entered into an open versus endoscopic randomised trial for class 6 venous disease in 1995. The trial was stopped after 39 patients had been entered because of the much greater incidence of wound complications in the open group (10/19 cf. 0/20 $p<0.001$). However, both groups had an 85% rate of ulcer healing. At a mean follow-up of 21 months (range 16 to 29 months) there had been no recurrences among those whose ulcers had originally healed [26].

In 1997, the North American SEPS study (NASEPS) was published [27]. They studied 155 SEPS operations carried out on 148 patients. There were no early deaths or problems with deep venous thrombosis. Wound infection occurred in 5% of the patients, most of whom had an open ulcer. Wound healing was 80% by six months post-surgery. They came to the conclusion that the procedure was safe, with wound infection being the only significant problem. Subsequently, a follow-up study was published which showed cumulative ulcer healing at one year of 88% [21]. It was also noted that post-phlebitic limbs had the highest recurrence rate (46% at two years).

A recent systematic review [3] identified 20 case series but only one randomised controlled trial of SEPS versus open surgery as discussed above (Pierik 1995) [26]. Combining the studies gave a total of 1031 patients who had 1140 limbs treated; 526 (46%) had active ulceration (C6), whilst 764 (67%) underwent additional venous procedures at the same time as SEPS.

The studies which described follow-up data were combined to give an ulcer healing rate of 40% by 30 days and 64% by 60 days. Subsequent recurrence was 13% during a mean follow-up of 21 months. In a later report of longer-term follow-up, although ulcer recurrence was higher in the post-thrombotic limbs, clinical improvement was still significant [28].

Conclusions

Venous ulceration places a tremendous burden on the patient and health services. The prognosis is poor with only 50% healed at four months [29], 20% remaining open after two years and 8% still unhealed at five years [30]. Duplex has provided us with more information about the dynamics of the venous system in these cases and from this, potential for surgical intervention. Endoscopic calf perforator surgery appears to now be a reliable and safe technique. However, the extent to which the correction of these perforators will be helpful in these patients in the long-term has yet to be established. Many of the patients operated on have additional procedures making analysis of the SEPS component of surgery more difficult. However, long-term ulcer healing does appear possible and the incidence of complications is acceptable and certainly markedly less than for an equivalent open procedure. Clinical series to date report healing and recurrence rates which favourably compare with the results of conservative management. Unfortunately, our understanding of the mechanisms underlying ulcer formation in chronic venous disease is still only very basic. With a greater knowledge of the pathophysiology we will be in a better position to anticipate those patients in whom disconnection of the perforating calf veins will be of benefit.

Key Summary

◆ Incompetent calf perforators are often associated with ankle ulceration.

◆ However, only a minority (<5%) of ankle ulcers are associated with incompetent calf perforators alone.

◆ Open perforator surgery is associated with high rates of infections and delayed wound healing.

◆ Calf perforating veins can be divided safely and effectively using the SEPS technique.

◆ SEPS can be combined with other forms of superficial venous surgery.

◆ The perforators should be marked with duplex prior to SEPS.

◆ SEPS is not recommended for routine varicose vein surgery.

◆ SEPS appears to improve ulcer healing rates in appropriate patients.

◆ There is a lack of randomised trials concerning SEPS and long-term ulcer healing rates.

References

1. Cockett FB, Jones DE. The ankle blow-out syndrome, a new approach to the varicose ulcer problem. *Lancet* 1953; 1(1): 17-23.
2. Nelzen O, Bergqvist D, Lindhagen A. Leg ulcer etiology - a cross-sectional population study. *J Vasc Surg* 1991; 14: 557-64.
3. Tenbrook JA, Jr., Iafrati MD, O'Donnell T F, Jr., Wolf MP, Hoffman SN, Pauker SG, *et al*. Systematic review of outcomes after surgical management of venous disease incorporating subfascial endoscopic perforator surgery. *J Vasc Surg* 2004; 39(3): 583-9.
4. Hyde GL, Litton TC, Hull DA. Long-term results of subfascial vein ligation for venous stasis disease. *Surg Gynecol Obstet* 1981; 153: 683-6.
5. Negus D, Friedgood A. The effective management of venous ulceration. *Br J Surg* 1983; 70: 623-7.
6. Silver D, Gleysteen JJ, Rhodes GR, Georgiade NG, Anlyan WG. Surgical treatment of the refractory postphlebitic ulcer. *Arch Surg* 1971; 103: 554-60.
7. Jamieson WG, DeRose G, Harris KA. Management of venous stasis ulcer: long-term follow-up. *Can J Surg* 1990; 33: 222-3.
8. Bowen FH. Subfascial ligation (Linton operation) of the perforating leg veins to treat post-thrombophlebitic syndrome. *Am Surg* 1975; 41(3): 148-51.
9. Beebe HG, Bergan JJ, Bergqvist D, Eklof B, Eriksson I, Goldman MP, *et al*. Classification and grading of chronic venous disease in the lower limbs. A consensus statement. *Eur J Vasc Endovasc Surg* 1996; 12(4): 487-91.
10. Albanese AR. Escoplage: a new surgical technique for the treatment of varicose veins in the legs. *J Cardiovasc Surg* 1965; 6: 491-4.
11. Edwards JM. Shearing operation for incompetent perforating veins. *Br J Surg* 1976; 63: 885-6.
12. Hauer G. Endoscopic subfascial discussion of perforating veins - preliminary report. *Vasa* 1985; 14(1): 59-61.
13. Fischer R. Surgical treatment of varicose veins; endoscopic treatment of incompetent Cockett veins. *Phlebology* 1989; 42: 1040-1.
14. Linton RR. The communicating veins of the lower leg and the operative technique for their ligation. *Ann Surg* 1938; 107: 582-93.
15. Cockett FB. The pathology and treatment of venous ulcers of the leg. *Br J Surg* 1955; 43(179): 260-78.
16. Mozes G, Gloviczki P, Menawat SS, Fisher DR, Carmichael SW, Kadar A. Surgical anatomy for endoscopic subfascial division of perforating veins. *J Vasc Surg* 1996; 24(5): 800-8.
17. Baron HC, Wayne MG, Santiago CA, Grossi R. Endoscopic subfascial perforator vein surgery for patients with severe, chronic venous insufficiency. *Vasc Endovasc Surg* 2004; 38(5): 439-42.
18. Bianchi C, Ballard JL, Abou-Zamzam AM, Teruya TH. Subfascial endoscopic perforator vein surgery combined with saphenous vein ablation: results and critical analysis. *J Vasc Surg* 2003; 38(1): 67-71.

19. Mendes RR, Marston WA, Farber MA, Keagy BA. Treatment of superficial and perforator venous incompetence without deep venous insufficiency: is routine perforator ligation necessary? *J Vasc Surg* 2003; 38(5): 891-5.

20. Iafrati MD, Pare GJ, O'Donnell TF, Estes J. Is the nihilistic approach to surgical reduction of superficial and perforator vein incompetence for venous ulcer justified? *J Vasc Surg* 2002; 36(6): 1167-74.

21. Gloviczki P, Bergan JJ, Rhodes JM, Canton LG, Harmsen S, Ilstrup DM. Mid-term results of endoscopic perforator vein interruption for chronic venous insufficiency: lessons learned from the North American subfascial endoscopic perforator surgery registry. The North American Study Group. *J Vasc Surg* 1999; 29(3): 489-502.

22. Rhodes JM, Gloviczki P, Canton LG, Rooke T, Lewis BD, Lindsey JR. Factors affecting clinical outcome following endoscopic perforator vein ablation. *Am J Surg* 1998; 176(2): 162-7.

23. Tawes RL, Wetter LA, Hermann GD, Fogarty TJ. Endoscopic technique for subfascial perforating vein interruption. *J Endovasc Surg* 1996; 3(4): 414-20.

24. Jugenheimer M, Junginger T. Endoscopic subfascial sectioning of incompetent perforating veins in treatment of primary varicosis. *World J Surg* 1992; 16(5): 971-5.

25. Pierik EG, Wittens CH, van Urk H. Subfascial endoscopic ligation in the treatment of incompetent perforating veins. *Eur J Vasc Endovasc Surg* 1995; 9(1): 38-41.

26. Pierik EG, van Urk H, Hop WC, Wittens CH. Endoscopic versus open subfascial division of incompetent perforating veins in the treatment of venous leg ulceration: a randomized trial. *J Vasc Surg* 1997; 26(6): 1049-54.

27. Gloviczki P, Bergan JJ, Menawat SS, Hobson RW, Kistner RL, Lawrence PF, *et al.* Safety, feasibility and early efficacy of subfascial endoscopic perforator surgery: a preliminary report from the North American registry. *J Vasc Surg* 1997; 25(1): 94-105.

28. Kalra M, Gloviczki P. Surgical treatment of venous ulcers: role of subfascial endoscopic perforator vein ligation. *Surg Clin North Am* 2003; 83(3): 671-705.

29. Skene AL, Smith JM, Dore CJ, Charlett A, Lewis JD. Venous leg ulcers: a prognostic index to predict time to healing. *Br Med J* 1992; 305(6862): 1119-21.

30. DaSilva A, Widmer LK, Martin H, Hall TH, Glaus L, Schneider M. Varicose veins and chronic venous insufficiency. *Vasa* 1974; 3(2): 118-25.

Chapter 11

Sclerotherapy for venules and their feeder veins

Marianne Vandendriessche MD FRCS (Belg)

Consultant Vascular Surgeon, Jan Palfyn Hospital, Gent, Belgium and London Vein Institute, UK

Introduction

Patients suffering from venous insufficiency seek advice for many reasons, including heaviness, tiredness, varicose eczema, ulceration, bleeding varices and looks. Cosmetic disfigurement can be the primary concern, or the only complaint. Especially in the private sector, looks and aesthetics are an important aspect. Treating patients for their varicose veins without being capable of dealing with the venules, will leave your patient dissatisfied.

Aetiology

Primary venules can be present without any other venous abnormality (CEAP I) [1]. They are more common in females and can appear suddenly at any stage during pregnancy (pregnant flares). Most venules are noticed at times of hormonal fluctuations, i.e. at the onset of puberty, with pregnancy, and at the menopause. Some skin types are more prone to the development of these venous flares, i.e. Mediterranean. There is often a hereditary tendency [2]. Venules may also be associated with an underlying venous problem (venous reflux and/or obstruction). These secondary venules must be differentiated from primary venules because the treatment will be different.

Diagnosis

A full history and clinical examination are necessary. A duplex ultrasound examination will differentiate primary venules from secondary venules by demonstrating the underlying venous problem. Venules may be the only abnormality complained of and seen during a brief clinical examination, but are in fact secondary to an underlying vein problem (Table 1) [3].

Table 1 Association of secondary venules with underlying vein problems.

Location of venules	Cause: incompetent vein
Medial malleolus	GSV
(ankle flare)	Lower leg perforator
Lateral malleolus	SSV
	Lateral perforator (from soleus)
Mid-calf	Mid-calf perforator (from gastrocnemius)
Front of lower leg	Paratibial perforator (from GSV)

Treatment

Treatment of secondary venules

Treatment of secondary venules alone without dealing with the underlying cause is unlikely to produce a satisfactory result. Often, persistent venules, causing frustration for the doctor and disappointment for the patient, are the result of a persisting underlying source of venous reflux (tributary, perforator or main trunk). Treatment of the primary venous reflux is therefore mandatory (by surgery, foam sclerotherapy, endovenous laser therapy [EVLT], radiofrequency closure [VNUS Closure®]). Reticular veins or feeder veins, related to patches of spider veins can be eliminated by phlebectomy when treating the larger veins.

Having dealt with the underlying reflux, the secondary venules will often diminish and may even disappear during the first few months after treatment, but if they persist they can then be successfully treated in a similar manner as for primary venules.

Treatment of primary venules

Sclerotherapy is the only effective method of treating dilated venules. The plan of treatment is shown in the algorithm (Figure 1). Several sessions may be necessary to completely eliminate all venules and feeder veins.

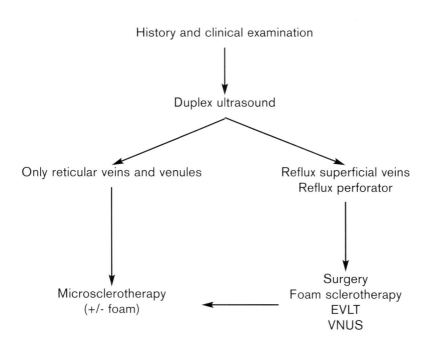

Figure 1 Treatment plan for microsclerotherapy.

The sclerosants used are loaded in 1ml syringes fitted with 30g needles and the effective drugs are listed in Table 2. The volume of sclerosant used at each site depends upon the extent of the patch of venules. Injecting too much sclerosant at a single site can cause telangiectatic matting. This reddish matting of minute venules, at the site of such injection is difficult to manage. Recently, the use of the sclerosant in the form of microfoam has been shown to be advantageous. However, only sclerosant with a detergent action can be converted to foam. This is applicable for polidocanol but not for glycerine.

Table 2 Preferred sclerosants used for the treatment of dilated venules and feeder veins.

Feeder veins	Polidocanol 1% +/- used as foam
(reticular veins)	(CH - Sclerovein, D-Aethoxysclerol)
Venules	Glycerine 72% +/- lignocaine
	Polidocanol 0.5%
	(CH - Sclerovein, D-Aethoxysclerol)

The use of polidocanol foam when injecting feeder veins allows it to spread further into the reticular veins and the venules [4, 5], and so a smaller volume of sclerosant is used. The treatment of venules with polidocanol foam injected directly into the venules has been claimed to be effective. The author's personal preference is a combined technique using polidocanol 1% (+/- microfoam produced by the Tessari method [6]) for the feeder veins (2-3mm diameter), and 72% glycerine for the venules, as this avoids complications and is very effective.

Aftercare

Appropriate compression is mandatory! When only treating feeder veins and venules a 30mmHg pressure stocking is applied. It is worn continually day and night, for five days and then only during the day for a further ten days. These stockings or tights are very elegant and cosmetically acceptable. During the winter this regime is easily accepted. When extensive venules and feeder veins are all treated at one session it may be advantageous to apply a compression bandage for the first five days, followed by stockings worn during the day for a further ten days [7]. Patients are reviewed after two weeks and small intravascular clots (if present) are aspirated (Table 3).

Table 3 Reasons for treating intravascular blood clots following microsclerotherapy.

- Elimination of the local pain
- Elimination of risk of subsequent pigmentation which can be permanent
- Prevention of recanalisation of feeder veins which is likely to result in failure

---

Complications of sclerotherapy

As with all treatment, complications are possible and so the practitioner must be fully aware and prepared to deal with them [8, 9]. If the treatment is applied with precision, serious complications (skin necrosis) are unlikely and minor complications are easily managed. The most severe complication which must be recognised and treated promptly, although fortunately extremely rare, is allergy and so appropriate equipment must be immediately available. All possible complications are listed in Table 4.

Instructions given to the patient

A brochure, describing the technique of microsclerotherapy is given to the patient at the initial consultation. All frequent complications are described and the need for several treatment sessions is clearly explained. Immediately following the first treatment session, the leg may appear bruised and this is clearly stated in the brochure. The cost is given.

Table 4 Possible complications of sclerotherapy.

Glycerine	
Allergy	None
Cutaneous	Matting (rare)
Others	Migraine
Polidocanol	
Allergy	Urticaria
	Bronchospasm
	Anaphylactic shock
Cutaneous	Pigmentation
	Matting
	Aseptic Abscess (perivenous injection)
	Skin necrosis (intra-arterial injection)
Others	Transient visual disorder
	Migraine

Patients are advised to look at the website for more details of the treatment, for alternative treatments, and to view 'before and after' pictures.

Other suggested treatments for management of dilated venules

Laser

Several different lasers have been promoted for the treatment of venules. Although extremely successful for the face and the chest, this method is not effective for the elimination of dilated venules on the legs.

Electrocoagulation

Electrocoagulation has been advocated but this method is ineffective and when venules are eliminated there is often significant local skin damage resulting in unsightly scars.

Miracle creams

In the lay press, creams are advertised for the treatment of dilated venules (spider veins) and are based on vitamins and claimed to be effective. None have been shown to have any effect and are often very expensive. The only preparations which have a possible application are camouflage creams but these are very temporary as they hide, but do not treat, the venules.

Conclusions

Dilated superficial veins and venules (primary or secondary) can successfully be treated by sclerotherapy (foam sclerotherapy combined with liquid sclerotherapy or liquid sclerotherapy only).

When properly performed by trained phlebologists the risks are minimal and the results optimal.

Key Summary

◆ Venules may be a minor but significant cosmetic problem.

◆ The development of venules is related to inherited skin types and hormone changes.

◆ Venules may be secondary to an underlying vein problem.

◆ If the underlying vein problem is not recognised, treatment will fail and the condition will be made worse.

◆ Therefore, any significant venous reflux must first be eliminated by surgery or perhaps by ultrasound-guided foam sclerotherapy.

◆ Reticular veins can be treated by sclerotherapy when treating the venules.

◆ Venules are eliminated by sclerotherapy using appropriate drugs.

◆ Compression is necessary and related to vessel size.

◆ Complications are minor and rare.

References

1. Eklof B, *et al.* Revision of the CEAP classification for chronic venous disorders: Consesus statement. *J Vasc Surg* 2004; 40: 1248-52.
2. Sadick NS. Predisposing factors of varicose and telangiectatic leg veins. *J Dermatol Surg Oncol* 1992; 18: 883-6.
3. Uhl JF, *et al.* Clinical and hemodynamic significance of corona phlebectatica in chronic venous disorders. *J Vasc Surg* 2005; 42: 1163-8.

4. Benigni JP, *et al.* Télangiectasies et varices réticulaires, traitement par la mousse. *Phlébologie* 1999; 52: 283-90.
5. Henriet JP. Experience durant trois années de la mousse de polidocanol dans le traitement des varices réticulaires et des varicosités. *Phlébologie* 1999; 52: 277-82.
6. Tessari L. Nouvelle technique d'obtention de la scléro-mousse. *Phlébologie* 2000; 53: 129.
7. Goldman MP. How to utilise compresssion after sclerotherapy. *Dermatol Surg* 2002; 28: 860-2.
8. Hobbs JT. Sclerosing and compression therapy for varicose veins - four decades of experience. In: *Trends in Vascular Surgery*. Pearce WH, Matsumura JS, Yao JST, Eds. Evanston: Greenwood Academic, 2006: 33-46.
9. Frullini A, Cavezzi A. Sclerosing foam in the treatment of varicose veins and teliangiectases: history and analysis of safety and complications. *Dermatol Surg* 2002; 28: 11-5.

Chapter 12
The prophylaxis and treatment of venous thrombo-embolism

Joseph A Caprini MD MS FACS RVT

Louis W. Biegler Professor of Surgery and Bioengineering, Department of Surgery,
Evanston Northwestern Healthcare, Evanston, Illinois, USA
Northwestern University Feinberg School of Medicine, Chicago, Illinois, USA and
Robert R. McCormick School of Engineering and Applied Sciences, Evanston, Illinois, USA

Introduction

Venous thrombo-embolism (VTE), a serious disease that encompasses deep venous thrombosis (DVT) and pulmonary embolism (PE), continues to be a significant cause of morbidity and mortality [1, 2]. As many as 145 individuals per 100,000 in the general population develop symptomatic DVT every year, and up to 69 individuals per 100,000 experience PE [3]. One-year mortality rates can be up to 21% for DVT and more than 50% for PE [4, 5]. Long-term complications of DVT of the lower extremity, including proximal or distal calf vein thrombosis, include post-thrombotic syndrome (PTS), resulting from chronic venous insufficiency to the affected limb, and recurrent VTE [6]. PTS is characterised by permanent vein damage, resulting in chronic leg swelling that worsens during the day and that may be accompanied by varicose veins, oedema, skin discoloration, and skin ulceration [6, 7]. PE can be classified as massive, which is often fatal and must be resolved immediately by thrombolysis, or non-massive, which is not immediately life-threatening and can be treated with anticoagulation. Long-term complications of PE include increased pulmonary artery pressure, pulmonary hypertension, and right-sided heart failure [8]. These serious, disabling, and sometimes fatal consequences of VTE underscore the importance of prevention in patients at risk.

VTE risk assessment

Risk for VTE should be assessed in all hospitalised patients. This practice is endorsed by the National Quality Forum (NQF), which published a consensus report on safe practices for better healthcare in 2003 [9]. NQF-endorsed safe practice #17 states that physicians should "evaluate each patient upon admission, and regularly thereafter, for the risk of developing DVT/VTE. Utilise clinically appropriate methods to prevent DVT/VTE." Risk assessment is required to stratify patients, according to overall VTE risk, to allow for optimal decision making regarding VTE prophylaxis, including modality, agent, and duration of prophylaxis [10]. Risk assessment can also be a useful aid in the diagnosis of VTE and may be used to guide decisions about the duration of treatment following an acute episode of VTE [10].

Risk factors

Because risk category placement is dependent on the presence of factors that influence the risk for VTE, identification of VTE risk factors is critical for the appropriate initiation of therapy [1]. There is a wide range of hereditary, medical, and surgical conditions that may increase the risk for VTE (Table 1), and the presence of multiple risk factors can cumulatively increase the risk for a thrombo-embolic event [11, 12]. Different patient populations have different risk for VTE. The prevalence of DVT without treatment is particularly high among patients who have undergone major orthopaedic surgery (40% to 84%) or who have experienced major trauma (30% to 70%) or a spinal cord injury (50% to 90%) [13]. The prevalence of VTE without treatment in general surgical patients is approximately 30% [14, 15]. The prevalence of asymptomatic DVT without treatment in general medical patients ranges from 5% to 15% [16-22]. A complete patient history is necessary to identify factors in the clinical setting, patient factors, and thrombophilic factors that put a patient at risk for VTE.

Risk assessment models (RAMs) have been developed by assigning weight to VTE risk factors (based on the risk for VTE that they confer to a patient) to determine a patient's total risk factor score. This score can help guide physicians in prescribing an optimal VTE prophylaxis regimen for each patient.

Table 1 Inherited, acquired, medical, and surgical risk factors for VTE [23-28].

Hereditary and acquired risk factors

- Lupus anticoagulant, anticardiolipin, and antiphospholipid antibodies
- Hyperhomocysteinaemia
- Dysfibrinogenaemia
- Myeloproliferative disorders
- Antithrombin deficiency
- Factor V Leiden (activated protein C resistance)
- Disseminated intravascular coagulation
- Polycythaemia vera
- Disorders of plasminogen and plasminogen activation

- Heparin-induced thrombocytopenia
- Protein C deficiency
- Protein S deficiency
- Hyperviscosity syndromes
- Prothrombin gene mutation 20210A
- Heparin cofactor II deficiency
- Primary thrombocytosis
- Elevated FVIII, IX, XI levels

Medical risk factors

- Age >40 years
- Prolonged immobility
- Prolonged confinement to bed or lower limb paralysis
- History of venous thrombo-embolism
- Cancer
- Myocardial infarction
- Stroke
- Cardiac dysfunction or congestive heart failure
- Acute respiratory failure

- Pregnancy
- Obesity
- Varicose veins
- Oestrogen use
- Inflammatory bowel disease
- Nephrotic syndrome
- Indwelling femoral vein catheter/central lines
- Pacemaker wires
- Sepsis
- Endothelial damage (of any cause)

Surgical risk factors

- Major surgery (especially involving the abdomen, pelvis or lower extremities)
- Trauma or fractures to the pelvis, hip, or lower extremities

- Total hip replacement
- Total knee replacement

Risk assessment models

Ideal risk assessment models should apply to all types of hospital patients and be quick and simple to use, based on factors easily identified from medical history and physical examination. Patients should be stratified according to overall risk level, and specific recommendations for appropriate thromboprophylaxis should be based on evidence from randomised controlled trials [29, 30]. Several RAMs that meet these criteria have been published [1, 29, 31]. Caprini and colleagues combined the strengths of available RAMs and drew on consensus documents to develop a simple, self-contained scoring system for risk stratification of both surgical and medical patients, based on clearly defined clinical settings and the presence of specified risk factors (Table 2) [10]. This RAM can be used to assign each patient a total risk factor score, which can then be used to categorise patients into one of four risk categories (low, moderate, high, and highest) [10]. An appropriate method of VTE prophylaxis can be chosen based on the level of risk, taking into consideration any contraindications to prophylaxis.

Kucher, Goldhaber and colleagues evaluated a RAM linked to a computerised system that alerted the responsible physician to a patient's increased risk for VTE [32]. The programme used eight common risk factors (cancer, prior VTE, hypercoagulability, major surgery, advanced age, obesity, bed rest, and the use of hormone replacement therapy or oral contraceptives) to determine each hospitalised patient's risk for VTE. Patients at increased risk were randomised to the electronic alert group or a control group. Significantly ($p<0.001$) more patients in the electronic alert group received mechanical or pharmacologic prophylaxis. At 90 days, 4.9% of patients in the electronic alert group experienced DVT or a PE compared with 8.2% of patients in the control group, a reduction of 41%. Goldhaber's results suggest that the use of RAMs to identify and treat patients at risk for VTE can significantly reduce the rate of VTE.

Selected highlights of VTE prophylaxis

2004 ACCP guidelines for VTE prophylaxis

Beginning in 1986 and at each three-year interval thereafter, the American College of Chest Physicians (ACCP) has published consensus

12 The prophylaxis and treatment of venous thrombo-embolism

Table 2 Proposed VTE RAM for surgical and medical patients (adapted from Caprini *et al* [10]).

Step 1: Exposing risk factors associated with clinical setting			
Each risk factor represents 1 point	Each risk factor represents 2 points	Each risk factor represents 3 points	Each risk factor represents 5 points
☐ Minor surgery	☐ Major surgery* ☐ Immobilising plaster cast ☐ Patients confined to bed >72 hours ☐ Central venous access ☐ Arthroscopic surgery	☐ Myocardial infarction ☐ Congestive heart failure ☐ Severe sepsis/ infection	☐ Elective major lower extremity arthroplasty ☐ Hip, pelvis, or leg fracture (<1 month) ☐ Stroke (<1 month) ☐ Multiple trauma (<1 month) ☐ Acute spinal cord injury (<1 month)

*Operations in which the dissection is important or that last longer than 45 minutes, including laparoscopic procedures.

Exposing risk factor score: ___

Step 2: Predisposing risk factors associated with patient

	Molecular	
Clinical setting	Inherited (3 points)	Acquired (3 points)
☐ Age 40 to 60 years (1 point) ☐ Pregnancy or postpartum (<1 month; 1 point) ☐ Varicose veins (1 point) ☐ Inflammatory bowel disease (1 point) ☐ Obesity (BMI >25; 1 point) ☐ Combined oral contraceptive/ hormonal replacement therapy (1 point) ☐ Age >60 years (2 points) ☐ Malignancy (2 points) ☐ Age >75 years (3 points) ☐ History of DVT/PE (3 points)	☐ Factor V Leiden/activated ☐ Antithrombin III deficiency ☐ Proteins C and S deficiency ☐ Dysfibrinogenaemia ☐ Homocysteinaemia ☐ 20210A prothrombin mutation	☐ Lupus anticoagulant ☐ Antiphospholipid antibodies ☐ Myeloproliferative disorders ☐ Disorders of plasminogen and plasmin activation ☐ Heparin-induced thrombocytopenia ☐ Hyperviscosity

Predisposing risk factor score: ___

Step 3: Total risk factor score (Exposing + Predisposing): ___

guidelines on appropriate VTE prophylaxis and treatment. These guidelines strictly adhere to an evidence-based approach and are often cited as standard of care [33]. The ACCP categorises patients according to the type of hospital service that is providing care and makes graded recommendations for each group with regard to the benefits and risks of specific options [1]. Table 3 details the different grades that are assigned and the rationale behind each grade.

General surgery

Table 4 summarises the 2004 ACCP recommendations for VTE prophylaxis in general surgery [1]. Two pharmacologic regimens, low-dose unfractionated heparin (LDUH) and low-molecular-weight heparins (LMWHs), are recommended (grade 1A) for use in moderate- and high-risk patients. High-risk doses (5000 U TID vs BID for LDUH and >3400 U QD vs ≤3400 U QD for LMWH) are recommended in high-risk patients. These recommendations are based on the results of randomised clinical trials demonstrating that both agents reduce the risk of both asymptomatic and symptomatic VTE in general surgery by at least 60% and have similar bleeding rates [1, 13, 15, 35-43]. No study reported a difference in the rate of symptomatic VTE between the two regimens [1].

Mechanical prophylaxis alone has not been well studied in general surgery; therefore, mechanical prophylaxis alone is only recommended in patients at high risk for bleeding (grade 1A) [1]. Studies have demonstrated lower rates of VTE with mechanical plus pharmacologic prophylaxis compared with pharmacologic alone [44-46]; therefore, in patients at the highest risk for VTE (those with multiple risk factors), mechanical prophylaxis (graduated compression stockings [GCS] or intermittent pneumatic compression [IPC]) in conjunction with pharmacologic prophylaxis is recommended (grade 1C+). Finally, extended prophylaxis (two to three weeks) with LMWH is recommended (grade 2A) in selected high-risk patients, such as those who have undergone major cancer surgery, based on data from three clinical trials [47-50].

At the time the 2004 ACCP guidelines were published, fondaparinux, the selective inhibitor of factor Xa, was not approved in the USA for use in general surgery and was, therefore, not given a recommendation.

Table 3 ACCP grades of recommendation for antithrombotic agents *.
Reproduced with permission from Guyatt et al [34].

Grade of recommendation	Clarity of risk/benefit	Methodological strength of supporting evidence	Implications
1A	Clear	RCTs without important limitations	Strong recommendation; can apply to most patients in most circumstances without reservation
1C+	Clear	No RCTs, but RCT results can be unequivocally extrapolated, or overwhelming evidence from observational studies	Strong recommendation; can apply to most patients in most circumstances
1B	Clear	RCTs with important limitations (inconsistent results, methodological flaws†)	Strong recommendation; likely to apply to most patients
1C	Clear	Observational studies	Intermediate-strength recommendation; may change when stronger evidence is available
2A	Unclear	RCTs without limitations	Intermediate-strength; best action may differ depending on circumstances or patient's societal values
2C+	Unclear	No RCTs but strong RCT results can be unequivocally extrapolated, or overwhelming evidence from observational studies	Weak recommendation; best action may differ depending on circumstances or patient's societal values
2B	Unclear	RCT with important limitations	Weak recommendation; alternatives likely better for some patients under some circumstances
2C	Unclear	Observational studies	Very weak recommendation; other alternatives may be equally reasonable

* Because studies in categories B and C are flawed, it is likely that most recommendations in these classes will be level 2. The following considerations will bear on whether the recommendation is Grade 1 or Grade 2: the magnitude and precision of the treatment effect; patients' risk of the target event being prevented; the nature of the benefit and the magnitude of the risk associated with treatment; variability in patient preferences; variability in regional resource availability and healthcare delivery practices; and cost considerations. Inevitably, weighing these considerations involves subjective judgment.
†These situations include RCTs with both lack of blinding and subjective outcomes, where the risk of bias in measurement of outcomes is high, or RCTs with large loss to follow-up.
RCT = randomised controlled trial

Table 4 ACCP VTE prophylaxis recommendations in general surgery [1].

Regimen	Low risk [1] (minor surgery, <40 years of age)	Moderate risk (minor surgery, 40-60 years of age or additional risk factors OR surgery, <40 years of age)	High risk (minor surgery, >60 years of age or additional risk factors OR surgery, >40 years of age or additional risk factors)	Highest risk (surgery with multiple risk factors)
LDUH (5000 U BID)	-	1A	-	-
LDUH (5000 U TID)	-	-	1A	1A
LMWH (≤3400 U QD)	-	1A	-	-
LMWH (>3400 U QD)	-	-	1A	1A
Extended LMWH (2-3 weeks)	-	-	2A[2]	2A[2]
Mechanical prophylaxis (GCS or IPC)	-	- [3]	- [3]	1C+[4]

1 The use of specific prophylaxis other than early and persistent mobilisation is not recommended in low-risk general surgery patients (grade 1C+).

2 In selected high-risk general surgery patients, including those who have undergone major cancer surgery, post-hospital discharge prophylaxis with LMWH is recommended.

3 In general surgery patients at moderate to high risk for VTE with a high risk of bleeding, the use of mechanical prophylaxis with properly fitted GCS or IPC, at least initially until the bleeding risk decreases, is recommended (grade 1A).

4 In high-risk general surgery patients with multiple risk factors, it is recommended that mechanical prophylaxis be combined with the use of GCS and/or IPC.

LMWH = low-molecular-weight heparin, LDUH = low-dose unfractionated heparin, IPC = intermittent pneumatic compression, GCS = graduated compression stockings, - = no specific recommendation made, IPC = Intermittent pneumatic compression, QD = daily, BID = twice per day, TID = three times per day

However, fondaparinux has since been approved in the USA for prophylaxis in abdominal surgical patients undergoing general anaesthesia for longer than 45 minutes, who are older than 40 years of age and have one of the following risk factors: neoplastic disease, obesity, chronic obstructive pulmonary disease, inflammatory bowel disease, history of DVT or PE, or congestive heart failure. In addition, it is indicated for abdominal surgical patients undergoing general anaesthesia lasting longer than 45 minutes who are older than 60 years of age with or without one or more of the risk factors listed above. This indication was based on two independent trials including one study demonstrating that postoperative fondaparinux (2.5mg daily) was at least as safe and effective as LMWH (5000 IU daily) in high-risk abdominal surgical patients [51]. In a subset analysis of this study in patients with cancer, fondaparinux significantly (p=0.02) reduced the incidence of VTE compared with LMWH, without increasing major bleeding. According to a published abstract on a trial with fondaparinux in patients undergoing abdominal surgery, IPC alone had a very low incidence of venographic VTE events (5.3%); however, IPC plus fondaparinux significantly reduced the incidence of venographic events to 1.7% (p=0.004) [46].

Orthopaedic surgery

Table 5 summarises the 2004 ACCP recommendations for VTE prophylaxis in orthopaedic surgery. All patients undergoing major orthopaedic surgery on a lower limb (total knee replacement [TKR], total hip replacement [THR], hip fracture surgery [HFS], or knee arthroscopy) are known to be at risk for VTE. Each surgery places the patient at a different risk for VTE. Data on which the recommendations are based were sufficient to recommend at least one prophylactic regimen (fondaparinux, LMWHs, or warfarin) supported by 1A evidence for short-term prophylaxis in THR, TKR, and HFS [1]. Reductions in prevalence of DVT associated with these anticoagulant regimens are summarised in Figure 1 [13, 52-55].

Table 5 ACCP VTE prophylaxis recommendations in orthopaedic surgery [1].

Regimen	Total hip replacement (≥10 d/28-35 d)	Total knee replacement [1] (≥10 d)	Knee arthroscopy (high risk) [6] (≥10 d)	Hip fracture surgery (≥10 d/28-35 d)
Fondaparinux [2]	1A/1C+	1A	-	1A/1A
LMWH [3]	1A/1A	1A	2B	1C+/1C+
Warfarin [4]	1A/1A	1A	-	2B/1C+
Mechanical prophylaxis	1A against [5]			1C+ if anticoagulant contraindicated
IPC		1B	-	
GCS		-		
VFP		1A against [5]		
Aspirin	1A against [5]	1A against [5]	-	1A against [5]
LDUH	1A against [5]	1A against [5]	-	1B/-

1 Extended prophylaxis in knee replacement is not presently recommended.

2 2.5mg started 6 to 8 hours postoperatively.

3 For hip replacement: high-risk dose started 12 hours pre- or postoperatively OR half usual high-risk dose 4 to 6 hours postoperatively continued next day at full dose. For knee replacement and hip fracture: usual high-risk dose.

4 Adjusted to INR 2.5 (range 2-3), started pre-operatively or evening after surgery.

5 Not recommended as sole prophylaxis.

6 Prophylaxis following surgery is only recommended in patients at high risk for VTE.

LMWH = low-molecular-weight heparin, LDUH = low-dose unfractionated heparin, IPC = intermittent pneumatic compression, GCS = graduated compression stockings, VFP = venous foot pump, - = no specific recommendation made

Mechanical prophylaxis alone was recommended as an alternative in TKR (grade 1B) and in HFS (grade 1C+) when anticoagulants are contra-indicated due to a high bleeding risk or as an adjunct to pharmacologic prophylaxis (grade 2A). It is also recommended (grade 1C+) that the proper use of, and optimal compliance with, the mechanical device is ensured. In addition, routine prophylactic use was not recommended (grade 2B) for use in patients undergoing knee arthroscopy who are not at increased risk for VTE (no pre-existing VTE risk factors, or surgery is not prolonged or complicated).

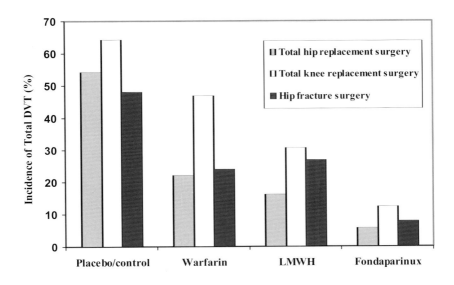

Figure 1 Reductions in DVT prevalence with VTE prophylaxis.

It was recommended (grade 1A) that the timing of the first dose of prophylaxis should be decided by weighing the effect of timing on risk of bleeding with its effect on the efficacy of each particular agent [1]. The effect of timing on the efficacy/bleeding ratio of each agent is not known; however, it is acceptable to use LMWHs either pre-operatively or postoperatively (grade 1A). Duration of prophylaxis in THR, TKR, and HFS was recommended to be at least ten days (grade 1A). Extended prophylaxis (up to 28 to 35 days) was recommended in THR and HFS (grade 1A). Fondaparinux was the only grade 1A recommended option for extended prophylaxis in HFS, and the grade 1A recommendations for extended prophylaxis in THR were LMWH and warfarin.

Medical patients

In acutely ill medical patients who have been admitted to hospital with congestive heart failure or severe respiratory disease, or who are confined to bed and have one or more additional risk factors, prophylaxis with LDUH or LMWH is strongly recommended (grade 1A). Several studies evaluated these agents in medical patients and demonstrated significant reductions in the relative risk of DVT by approximately 70% compared with placebo, without increased risk of bleeding [16-20, 22]. In the most recent study, the PREVENT trial, LMWH significantly reduced the incidence of VTE by nearly 50% [22]. Of five studies that compared LDUH and LMWH in medical patients, four failed to find significant differences in DVT rates or bleeding between agents [56-59]. One study reported a significantly lower incidence of DVT with 40mg LMWH QD compared with 5000 U LDUH TID (15.6% vs 22.1%, p=0.04) [60].

Fondaparinux is not approved in the USA for use in medical patients; however, it has been shown to significantly (p=0.029) reduce the incidence of both VTE and fatal PE by nearly 50% compared with placebo, without increased major bleeding, in hospitalised patients with acute medical illness [61]. All of these agents (LDUH, LMWH and fondaparinux) significantly reduce the incidence of VTE in medical patients when compared with placebo. Thus, it is no longer valid not to use VTE prophylaxis in this patient population.

Mechanical prophylaxis (GCS or IPC) is recommended (grade 1C+) in medical patients with risk factors for VTE and in whom there is a contra-indication to anticoagulant prophylaxis. Although no randomised clinical trials have evaluated mechanical prophylaxis alone in medical patients, a recently completed trial in general surgery in the USA demonstrated a low incidence of VTE (5.3%) with IPC alone in moderate-risk patients and has provided an impetus for their use in this patient population [46]. Another recent trial in the prevention of VTE in stroke patients showed superior efficacy for the combination of anti-embolism stockings plus IPC compared with stockings [62].

Advantages and disadvantages of methods of VTE prophylaxis

Although mechanical methods of prophylaxis are attractive options in patients who have a high risk of bleeding, practical limitations include a lack of standardisation of the quality of the stockings, difficulty with fitting patients with unusual limb sizes or shapes, and poor compliance with their use by both healthcare providers and patients [63, 64]. The different available pharmacologic agents for VTE prophylaxis are compared in Table 6. The biggest advantage of warfarin is oral administration. Additional advantages include low cost, reversal of effects by vitamin K, no dose adjustment required with renal failure, and a slightly reduced risk of surgical-site bleeding and wound haematoma. Disadvantages include delayed onset of action, monitoring requirements, a common failure to achieve the desired international normalised ratio (INR), many dietary and drug interactions, a contraindication in patients at risk for bleeding, and a bleeding risk with extended prophylaxis.

LDUH was the first pharmacologic agent widely investigated for the prevention of VTE and has a long history of use. Other advantages of LDUH are reversal by protamine sulphate and low cost relative to LMWH and fondaparinux. A limitation of LDUH is its association (up to a 5% incidence) with heparin-induced thrombocytopenia (HIT), an antibody-mediated process characterised by a dramatic drop in platelets [77-79]. HIT can result in significant morbidity, including limb ischaemia resulting in limb loss and is associated with a mortality rate of 12% to 23% [80, 81]. HIT is associated with all heparins (LDUH and LMWHs), although it is more frequent with LDUH, and use of heparins should be avoided in patients with HIT or a history of HIT [77, 82]. Additional disadvantages of LDUH include intravenous administration requiring hospitalisation and a short half-life (half an hour to two hours) relative to other anticoagulants, necessitating more frequent dosing. However, a short half-life can sometimes be an advantage in the case of bleeding complications or for the management of patients with renal failure.

Clinical advantages of LMWH over LDUH include once-daily, subcutaneous administration, and a lower risk of HIT [77]. LMWHs also carry a risk for HIT and should not be used in patients with HIT or a history of HIT [37, 43, 78, 83]. Additional advantages include a higher anti-Xa activity compared with antithrombin activity, better bioavailability at low doses, no monitoring required, and a longer half-life (four hours), allowing for once-daily dosing in some patients. However, a long half-life can sometimes be a disadvantage in the case of bleeding complications or renal failure. It has also been suggested that survival may be increased in patients with cancer, particularly those at early stages of malignancy, who receive

Table 6 Therapeutic modalities for the prevention and/or treatment of VTE [1, 12, 65-76].

Agent	Indications for use	Perceived advantages	Perceived disadvantages	Adverse effects (incidence)
Warfarin	• Prophylaxis and/or treatment of VTE and its extension, and PE	• Oral administration • No dose adjustment required with renal failure • Effects neutralised by vitamin K • Slightly reduced risk for surgical-site bleeding and wound haematoma, compared with LMWH in THR and TKR	• Regular monitoring is required due to its narrow therapeutic window • Patients often fail to achieve therapeutic INR ranges • Delayed onset of action (at least 3 days) • Increased bleeding during extended prophylaxis • Many drug and dietary interactions	• Major bleeding (2%) • Skin necrosis (<0.1%)
LDUH	• Prophylaxis and treatment of VTE and its extension • DVT and PE prophylaxis in patients undergoing major abdominothoracic surgery or who for other reasons are at risk of developing thrombo-embolic disease (in a low-dose regimen)	• Extensive clinical experience • Immediate onset/offset of action • Effects neutralised with protamine sulphate • No dose adjustment required in patients with renal failure • Inexpensive	• Low bioavailability (28.6% SC), short half-life (0.5-3 hours), non-specific binding, and rapid clearance • Intravenous administration • Therapeutic monitoring of aPTT and frequent dose adjustments are required • Prolongs INR • Contraindicated in patients with severe thrombocytopenia • HIT	• Major bleeding (0%-7%) • Thrombocytopenia (0%-30%) • HIT (1%-5%) • Wound haematomas/infections (1%-4%) • Heparin-induced osteopenia /osteoporosis (30% with prolonged use)

Continued:

Agent	Indications for use	Perceived advantages	Perceived disadvantages	Adverse effects (incidence)
LMWHs	• VTE prophylaxis (enoxaparin and dalteparin only)	• 81%-100% bioavailability, long half-life (1.7-7 hrs), and predictable dose response	• Dose adjustment required in patients with renal failure (CrCl <30mL/min) or increased BMI	• Major bleeding (1%-4%) • Thrombocytopenia (<1%-3%) • HIT (lower rates than seen with LDUH)
Enoxaparin sodium	- THR during and following hospital	• Laboratory monitoring not required in most patients	• May be less effective than LDUH in patients with a high BMI when given QD	• Wound haematomas/infections (2%-3%)
Dalteparin sodium	- TKR (enoxaparin only) - Abdominal surgery patients at risk for thrombo-embolic complications	• Effects partially neutralised with protamine sulphate • QD dosing • SC administration	• May require anti-Xa activity monitoring in selected patients	Heparin-induced osteopenia/ osteoporosis (with prolonged use)
Tinzaparin sodium	- Medical patients at risk for thrombo-embolic complications due to acute illness • VTE treatment (enoxaparin and tinzaparin only): - Inpatient treatment of acute DVT with or without PE when administered in conjunction with warfarin - Outpatient treatment of DVT without PE when administered in conjunction with warfarin (enoxaparin only)	• Survival benefit in patients with cancer	• Therapeutic range depends on once vs twice daily administration	

Continued:

Table 6 *continued:*

Agent	Indications for use	Perceived advantages	Perceived disadvantages	Adverse effects (incidence)
Fondaparinux sodium	• VTE prophylaxis: - Hip fracture surgery, including extended prophylaxis - THR and TKR - Abdominal surgery with risk of thrombo-embolic complications • VTE treatment: - Acute DVT when administered in conjunction with warfarin - Acute PE when administered in conjunction with warfarin when initial therapy is administered in the hospital	• 100% bioavailability, lack of non-specific binding, and long half-life (17 hours) • No evidence of HIT to date • QD dosing • SC administration • Can be administered on outpatient basis • Bleeding similar to LDUH and LMWHs • Improved wound healing compared with LMWHs	• Contraindicated in patients with severe renal impairment (CrCl <30mL/min) • Contraindicated for prophylaxis in orthopaedic surgery in patients weighing <50kg • Long half-life • No reversal agent	• Major bleeding (1%-3%)

VTE = venous thrombo-embolism, DVT = deep venous thrombosis, PE = pulmonary embolism, LDUH = low-dose unfractionated heparin, LMWH = low-molecular-weight heparin, THR = total hip replacement, TKR = total knee replacement, HIT = heparin-induced thrombocytopenia, SC = subcutaneous, aPTT = activated partial thromboplastin time, INR = international normalised ratio, QD = once daily, BID = twice daily, CrCl = creatinine clearance

LMWH compared with LDUH, although the reason for this is not clear [84-87]. Disadvantages of LMWHs include renal excretion (precluding use in patients with renal failure), increased cost relative to LDUH, and incomplete reversal by protamine sulphate [88].

Fondaparinux is a novel synthetic pentasaccharide [89]. Because factor Xa inhibitors are a new class of agents, they do not have as strong a history of clinical use as LDUH and LMWH. However, fondaparinux has demonstrated similar efficacy in patients undergoing general surgery [51] and greater efficacy than LMWH in VTE prophylaxis following total joint replacement [53, 54] and hip fracture surgery [52]. An advantage of fondaparinux is that, unlike LDUH and LMWH, it has not been associated with HIT and can be used in patients with HIT or a history of HIT. In addition, fondaparinux is administered subcutaneously and has a 17-hour half-life, which allows for convenient, once-daily dosing, but is contraindicated for prophylaxis in patients weighing less than 50kg or renally impaired patients (creatinine clearance <30mL/min). Further, because fondaparinux does not interfere with thrombin binding, it has no negative effect on wound healing. Although the long half-life allows for convenient dosing, it can sometimes be a disadvantage in the case of bleeding complications. Fondaparinux is renally excreted and should not be used in patients with renal failure.

Selected highlights of VTE treatment with anticoagulation

2004 ACCP recommendations [71, 90]

ACCP recommendations for the management of VTE are summarised in Table 7 [71]. The currently recommended approach for treatment of acute DVT of the leg and acute non-massive PE is to start LDUH or LMWH and warfarin together upon diagnosis, and to discontinue heparin when the INR is stable and >2.0 (grade 1A). For patients with a high clinical suspicion of DVT or PE, treatment with anticoagulants while awaiting the outcome of diagnostic tests is recommended (grade 1C+) [71]. Although safety and efficacy with LDUH and LMWH in the treatment of DVT and PE are similar [91-96], LMWH is recommended over LDUH for DVT (outpatient treatment when possible [grade 1C] and inpatient treatment when

Table 7 ACCP recommendations for VTE treatment.

Regimen	Initial treatment of acute DVT	Long-term treatment of acute DVT			Initial treatment of acute non-massive PE	Long-term treatment of acute PE		
		Idiopathic[8]	Transient risk factor	Cancer[9]		Idiopathic[8]	Transient risk factor	Cancer[9]
IV LDUH[1]	1A[3,4]	-	-	-	1A[3]	-	-	-
SC LDUH[1]	1A[5]	-	-	-	-	-	-	-
LMWH[1]	1A (over LDUH)[6]	-	-	1A, 3-6 months	1A (over LDUH)	-	-	1A, 3-6 months
Warfarin (with heparin)[2]	1A[7]	1A, 6-12 months	1A, 3 months	-	1A[7]	1A, 6-12 months	1A, 3 months	-

1 Recommended duration of initial treatment is at least 5 days (grade 1C).

2 Dose should be adjusted to maintain a target INR of 2.5 (range, 3.1 to 4.0, grade 1A).

3 Administered by continuous infusion with dose adjustment to achieve and maintain an aPTT prolongation corresponding to plasma heparin levels from 0.3 to 0.7 IU/mL anti-Xa activity by the amidolytic assay (grade 1C+).

4 Recommended over LMWH in patients with severe renal failure (grade 2C).

5 Recommended initial dose is 35,000 U/24 h, with subsequent dosing to maintain the aPTT in the therapeutic range (grade 1C+).

6 Recommended over LDUH as an outpatient if possible (grade 1C), and as an inpatient if necessary (grade 1A).

7 Initiation of warfarin together with LMWH or LDUH on the first treatment day with discontinuation of heparin when the INR is stable and >2.0 is recommended (grade 1A).

8 Should be considered for indefinite anticoagulant therapy (grade 2A).

9 Anticoagulant therapy recommended indefinitely or until the cancer is resolved (grade 1C).

DVT = deep venous thrombosis, PE = pulmonary embolism, IV = intravenous, SC = subcutaneous, LDUH = low-dose unfractionated heparin, LMWH = low-molecular-weight heparin, aPTT = activated partial thromboplastin time, - = no recommendation made necessary [grade 1A]) and non-massive PE (grade 1A). This is primarily due to convenience of administration and cost savings associated with outpatient therapy or early hospital discharge [92, 97, 98].

Since the 2004 ACCP guidelines were published, fondaparinux (5.0, 7.5, or 10.0mg once daily in patients weighing <50kg, 50-100kg, or >100kg, respectively) has been shown to be at least as effective as LMWH (1mg/kg twice daily) for the initial treatment of acute DVT [99], and as effective as LDUH (continuous IV, ratio of the activated partial thromboplastin time [aPTT] to a control value, 1.5 to 2.5) for the initial treatment of acute PE, without increasing the risk for major bleeding [100].

For DVT, routine thrombolysis with thrombolytics or catheter-directed thrombolysis, including venous thrombectomy, is not recommended (grade 1A), except in selected patients at risk for limb loss. In PE, thrombolytics are not recommended (grade 1C) except in haemodynamically unstable patients (grade 2B). Catheter extraction or fragmentation and pulmonary embolectomy are not recommended (grade 1C), except in selected highly compromised patients who are unable to receive thrombolytic therapy or whose critical status does not allow sufficient time to infuse thrombolytic therapy (grade 2C). Vena caval interruption is not recommended for initial treatment of VTE (grade 1A), except in patients with a contraindication for anticoagulation or with recurrent VTE, despite anticoagulation (grade 2C).

Warfarin is recommended for long-term treatment of acute VTE over other treatment options, except in the case of patients with cancer, when LMWH is recommended based on studies showing greater efficacy over warfarin [101, 102]. For patients with cancer, the recommended duration is three to six months with LMWH (grade 1A), with a grade 1C recommendation for treatment indefinitely or until the cancer is resolved. Treatment indefinitely (grade 2C) or for 12 months (grade 1C+) is recommended in patients with a first episode of VTE who have documented antiphospholipid antibodies or two or more thrombophilic conditions (e.g. combined factor V Leiden and prothrombin 20210 gene mutations). In patients with a first episode of VTE and documented deficiency of antithrombin, protein C, or protein S or the factor V Leiden or prothrombin 20210 gene mutation, homocysteinemia, or high factor VIII levels, treatment is recommended for six to 12 months (grade 1A) or indefinitely (grade 2C). Recommendations for duration of treatment assign a relatively high value to preventing recurrent thrombo-embolic events and a relatively low value to bleeding and cost.

Advantages and disadvantages of methods of VTE treatment

The advantages and disadvantages of the pharmacologic anticoagulants are summarised in Table 6. Some advantages and disadvantages specific to VTE treatment will be discussed. With IV LDUH, anti-Xa activity must be monitored to determine the dose required to achieve and maintain therapeutic aPTT. In contrast, routine monitoring with anti-factor Xa level measurements are not required with LMWH (grade 1A) or fondaparinux. In addition, LMWH and fondaparinux can be used on an outpatient basis, which can result in significant cost savings. A limitation of LMWH is that it is not well tested in massive PE; thus, the indication for LMWH in the USA is limited to the inpatient or outpatient treatment of DVT with or without PE in conjunction with warfarin and not for PE alone. In contrast, fondaparinux has been tested in PE alone and is indicated for the treatment of PE.

Precautions

Any drug that is renally excreted should be used with caution in renally impaired patients. Both LMWH and fondaparinux are renally excreted. Because exposure of LMWH is significantly increased in patients with severe renal impairment (creatinine clearance <30mL/min), a dosage adjustment is recommended for therapeutic and prophylactic dosage ranges. No dosage adjustment is recommended in patients with moderate (creatinine clearance 30-50mL/min) and mild (creatinine clearance 50-80mL/min) renal impairment. Fondaparinux should be used with caution in patients with moderate renal impairment and is contraindicated in patients with severe renal impairment.

Over 20 case reports of spinal haematoma and paralysis have been reported with the use of LMWH in patients receiving neuraxial anaesthesia [103], ultimately leading to an FDA-mandated 'black box' warning. Thus, caution is recommended regarding the use of antithrombotic drugs in patients having spinal puncture or placement of an epidural catheter (evidence Grade 1C+). The current ACCP guidelines outline some precautions:

◆ if using warfarin, continuous epidural catheterisation should not be used for longer than one to two days due to unpredictable anticoagulant effects, and the INR should be less than 1.5 at the time of catheter removal;
◆ prophylactic LMWH can be given with an epidural catheter in place but the drug must be stopped for 12 hours with a twice-daily dose and 24 hours with a once-daily dose before removing the catheter, and one must wait two hours before giving the next dose;
◆ when an epidural is used, fondaparinux should not be given until the epidural catheter has been removed for at least two hours and should not be administered to patients receiving continuous epidural spinal block, due to presently insufficient safety data;
◆ neuraxial blockade should generally be avoided in patients with clinical bleeding disorders;
◆ insertion of the spinal needle in patients receiving anticoagulants or platelet inhibitors should be delayed until medication effects are minimal;
◆ prophylaxis should be delayed if a haemorrhagic aspirate (bloody tap) is noted during initial needle placement;
◆ removal of epidural catheters should occur when anticoagulant effects are minimal; and
◆ anticoagulant prophylaxis should be delayed for at least two hours after spinal needle placement or catheter removal.

Conclusions

VTE is a common, serious condition that can be disabling and sometimes fatal. The consequences of VTE underscore the importance of prevention in patients at risk. Risk assessment is required in all patients undergoing general or orthopaedic surgery and in all hospitalised patients. Risk assessment can guide decisions for prophylaxis and treatment of VTE, and can result in improved outcomes.

Key Summary

◆ Venous thrombo-embolism is a serious disorder causing significant morbidity and mortality.

◆ The long-term consequences of this disease are generally unappreciated and unrecognised.

◆ Thrombosis prophylaxis is vastly underused, particularly in the medically ill patient.

◆ Individual patient risk assessment should guide the type, duration and intensity of thrombosis prophylaxis according to the level of patient risk.

References

1. Geerts WH, Pineo GF, Heit JA, Bergqvist D, Lassen MR, Colwell CW, *et al.* Prevention of venous thromboembolism: the Seventh ACCP Conference on Antithrombotic and Thrombolytic Therapy. *Chest* 2004;126(3 Suppl): 338S-400S.
2. Anderson FA, Jr., Wheeler HB, Goldberg RJ, Hosmer DW, Patwardhan NA, Jovanovic B, *et al.* A population-based perspective of the hospital incidence and case-fatality rates of deep vein thrombosis and pulmonary embolism. The Worcester DVT Study. *Arch Intern Med* 1991; 151(5): 933-8.
3. Silverstein MD, Heit JA, Mohr DN, Petterson TM, O'Fallon WM, Melton LJ, 3rd. Trends in the incidence of deep vein thrombosis and pulmonary embolism: a 25-year population-based study. *Arch Intern Med* 1998; 158(6): 585-93.
4. Heit JA, Silverstein MD, Mohr DN, Petterson TM, O'Fallon WM, Melton LJ, 3rd. Predictors of survival after deep vein thrombosis and pulmonary embolism: a population-based, cohort study. *Arch Intern Med* 1999; 159(5): 445-53.
5. Kniffin WD, Jr., Baron JA, Barrett J, Birkmeyer JD, Anderson FA, Jr. The epidemiology of diagnosed pulmonary embolism and deep venous thrombosis in the elderly. *Arch Intern Med* 1994; 154(8): 861-6.
6. Prandoni P, Lensing AW, Cogo A, Cuppini S, Villalta S, Carta M, *et al.* The long-term clinical course of acute deep venous thrombosis. *Ann Intern Med* 1996; 125(1): 1-7.
7. Prandoni P, Villalta S, Bagatella P, Rossi L, Marchiori A, Piccioli A, *et al.* The clinical course of deep-vein thrombosis. Prospective long-term follow-up of 528 symptomatic patients. *Haematologica* 1997; 82(4): 423-8.
8. Goldhaber SZ. Pulmonary embolism. *N Engl J Med* 1998; 339(2): 93-104.

9. National Quality Forum. Safe practices for better healthcare: a consensus report. Washington DC; 2003.

10. Caprini JA, Arcelus JI, Reyna JJ. Effective risk stratification of surgical and nonsurgical patients for venous thromboembolic disease. *Semin Hematol* 2001; 38(2 Suppl 5): 12-9.

11. Rosendaal FR. Venous thrombosis: a multicausal disease. *Lancet* 1999; 353(9159): 1167-73.

12. Turpie AG, Chin BS, Lip GY. ABC of antithrombotic therapy: venous thromboembolism: treatment strategies. *Br Med J* 2002; 325(7370): 948-50.

13. Geerts WH, Heit JA, Clagett GP, Pineo GF, Colwell CW, Anderson FA, Jr., et al. Prevention of venous thromboembolism. *Chest* 2001; 119(Suppl 1): 132S-175S.

14. Kakkar VV, Corrigan TP, Fossard DP. Prevention of fatal postoperative pulmonary embolism by low doses of heparin. An international multicentre trial. *Lancet* 1975; 2(7924): 45-51.

15. Collins R, Scrimgeour A, Yusuf S, Peto R. Reduction in fatal pulmonary embolism and venous thrombosis by perioperative administration of subcutaneous heparin. Overview of results of randomized trials in general, orthopedic, and urologic surgery. *N Engl J Med* 1988; 318(18): 1162-73.

16. Gallus AS, Hirsh J, Tutle RJ, Trebilcock R, O'Brien SE, Carroll JJ, et al. Small subcutaneous doses of heparin in prevention of venous thrombosis. *N Engl J Med* 1973; 288(11): 545-51.

17. Belch JJ, Lowe GD, Ward AG, Forbes CD, Prentice CR. Prevention of deep vein thrombosis in medical patients by low-dose heparin. *Scott Med J* 1981; 26(2): 115-7.

18. Cade JF. High risk of the critically ill for venous thromboembolism. *Crit Care Med* 1982; 10(7): 448-50.

19. Dahan R, Houlbert D, Caulin C, Cuzin E, Viltart C, Woler M, et al. Prevention of deep vein thrombosis in elderly medical in-patients by a low molecular weight heparin: a randomized double-blind trial. *Haemostasis* 1986; 16(2): 159-64.

20. Samama MM, Cohen AT, Darmon JY, Desjardins L, Eldor A, Janbon C, et al. A comparison of enoxaparin with placebo for the prevention of venous thromboembolism in acutely ill medical patients. Prophylaxis in Medical Patients with Enoxaparin Study Group. *N Engl J Med* 1999; 341(11): 793-800.

21. Oger E, Bressollette L, Nonent M, Lacut K, Guias B, Couturaud F, et al. High prevalence of asymptomatic deep vein thrombosis on admission in a medical unit among elderly patients. *Thromb Haemost* 2002; 88(4): 592-7.

22. Leizorovicz A, Cohen AT, Turpie AG, Olsson CG, Vaitkus PT, Goldhaber SZ. Randomized, placebo-controlled trial of dalteparin for the prevention of venous thromboembolism in acutely ill medical patients. *Circulation* 2004; 110(7): 874-9.

23. Anderson FA, Jr., Wheeler HB, Goldberg RJ, Hosmer DW, Forcier A. The prevalence of risk factors for venous thromboembolism among hospital patients. *Arch Intern Med* 1992; 152(8): 1660-4.

24. Rosendaal FR. Risk factors for venous thrombotic disease. *Thromb Haemost* 1999; 82(2): 610-9.

25. Heit JA, O'Fallon WM, Petterson TM, Lohse CM, Silverstein MD, Mohr DN, et al. Relative impact of risk factors for deep vein thrombosis and pulmonary embolism: a population-based study. *Arch Intern Med* 2002; 162(11): 1245-8.

26. Anderson FA, Jr., Spencer FA. Risk factors for venous thromboembolism. *Circulation* 2003; 107(23 Suppl 1): 16-9.

27. Thromboembolic Risk Factors (THRIFT) Consensus Group. Risk of and prophylaxis for venous thromboembolism in hospital patients. *Br Med J* 1992; 305(6853): 567-74.

28. Alikhan R, Cohen AT, Combe S, Samama MM, Desjardins L, Eldor A, *et al.* Risk factors for venous thromboembolism in hospitalized patients with acute medical illness: analysis of the MEDENOX Study. *Arch Intern Med* 2004; 164(9): 963-8.

29. Second Thromboembolic Risk Factors (THRiFT II) Consensus Group. Risk of and prophylaxis for venous thromboembolism in hospital patients. *Phlebology* 1998; 13: 87-97.

30. Verstraete M. Prophylaxis of venous thromboembolism. *Br Med J* 1997; 314(7074): 123-5.

31. Prevention of venous thromboembolism. International Consensus Statement (guidelines according to scientific evidence). *Int Angiol* 1997; 16(1): 3-38.

32. Kucher N, Koo S, Quiroz R, Cooper JM, Paterno MD, Soukonnikov B, *et al.* Electronic alerts to prevent venous thromboembolism among hospitalized patients. *N Engl J Med* 2005; 352(10): 969-77.

33. Tapson VF. The evolution and impact of the American College of Chest Physicians consensus statement on antithrombotic therapy. *Clin Chest Med* 2003; 24(1): 139-51.

34. Guyatt G, Schunemann HJ, Cook D, Jaeschke R, Pauker S. Applying the grades of recommendation for antithrombotic and thrombolytic therapy: the Seventh ACCP Conference on Antithrombotic and Thrombolytic Therapy. *Chest* 2004; 126(3 Suppl): 179S-187S.

35. Clagett GP, Reisch JS. Prevention of venous thromboembolism in general surgical patients. Results of meta-analysis. *Ann Surg* 1988; 208(2): 227-40.

36. Mismetti P, Laporte S, Darmon JY, Buchmuller A, Decousus H. Meta-analysis of low molecular weight heparin in the prevention of venous thromboembolism in general surgery. *Br J Surg* 2001; 88(7): 913-30.

37. Kakkar VV, Cohen AT, Edmonson RA, Phillips MJ, Cooper DJ, Das SK, *et al.* Low molecular weight versus standard heparin for prevention of venous thromboembolism after major abdominal surgery. The Thromboprophylaxis Collaborative Group. *Lancet* 1993; 341(8840): 259-65.

38. Nurmohamed MT, Verhaeghe R, Haas S, Iriarte JA, Vogel G, van Rij AM, *et al.* A comparative trial of a low molecular weight heparin (enoxaparin) versus standard heparin for the prophylaxis of postoperative deep vein thrombosis in general surgery. *Am J Surg* 1995; 169(6): 567-71.

39. Bergqvist D, Burmark US, Frisell J, Hallbook T, Lindblad B, Risberg B, *et al.* Low molecular weight heparin once daily compared with conventional low-dose heparin twice daily. A prospective double-blind multicentre trial on prevention of postoperative thrombosis. *Br J Surg* 1986; 73(3): 204-8.

40. Bergqvist D, Matzsch T, Burmark US, Frisell J, Guilbaud O, Hallbook T, *et al.* Low molecular weight heparin given the evening before surgery compared with conventional low-dose heparin in prevention of thrombosis. *Br J Surg* 1988; 75(9): 888-91.

41. Efficacy and safety of enoxaparin versus unfractionated heparin for prevention of deep vein thrombosis in elective cancer surgery: a double-blind randomized multicentre trial with venographic assessment. ENOXACAN Study Group. *Br J Surg* 1997; 84(8): 1099-103.

42. McLeod RS, Geerts WH, Sniderman KW, Greenwood C, Gregoire RC, Taylor BM, *et al*. Subcutaneous heparin versus low-molecular-weight heparin as thromboprophylaxis in patients undergoing colorectal surgery: results of the Canadian colorectal DVT prophylaxis trial: a randomized, double-blind trial. *Ann Surg* 2001; 233(3): 438-44.

43. Koch A, Bouges S, Ziegler S, Dinkel H, Daures JP, Victor N. Low molecular weight heparin and unfractionated heparin in thrombosis prophylaxis after major surgical intervention: update of previous meta-analyses. *Br J Surg* 1997; 84(6): 750-9.

44. Amaragiri SV, Lees TA. Elastic compression stockings for prevention of deep vein thrombosis. *Cochrane Database Syst Rev* 2000; (3): CD001484.

45. Ramos R, Salem BI, De Pawlikowski MP, Coordes C, Eisenberg S, Leidenfrost R. The efficacy of pneumatic compression stockings in the prevention of pulmonary embolism after cardiac surgery. *Chest* 1996; 109(1): 82-5.

46. Turpie AG, Bauer KA, Caprini J, Comp PC, Gent M, Muntz J. Fondaparinux combined with intermittent pneumatic compression (IPC) versus IPC alone in the prevention of VTE after major abdominal surgery: results of the APOLLO study [abstract]. *J Thromb Haemost* 2005; 3(Suppl 1): Abstract P1046.

47. Lausen I, Jensen R, Jorgensen LN, Rasmussen MS, Lyng KM, Andersen M, *et al*. Incidence and prevention of deep venous thrombosis occurring late after general surgery: randomised controlled study of prolonged thromboprophylaxis. *Eur J Surg* 1998; 164(9): 657-63.

48. Bergqvist D, Agnelli G, Cohen AT, Eldor A, Nilsson PE, Le Moigne-Amrani A, *et al*. Duration of prophylaxis against venous thromboembolism with enoxaparin after surgery for cancer. *N Engl J Med* 2002; 346(13): 975-80.

49. Rasmussen MS. Preventing thromboembolic complications in cancer patients after surgery: a role for prolonged thromboprophylaxis. *Cancer Treat Rev* 2002; 28(3): 141-4.

50. Rasmussen MS, Willie-Jorgensen P, Jorgensen LN. Prolonged thromboprophylaxis with low molecular weight heparin (dalteparin) following major abdominal surgery for malignancy [abstract]. *Blood* 2003; 102: 56a.

51. Agnelli G, Bergqvist D, Cohen AT, Gallus AS, Gent M. Randomized clinical trial of postoperative fondaparinux versus perioperative dalteparin for prevention of venous thromboembolism in high-risk abdominal surgery. *Br J Surg* 2005; 92(10): 1212-20.

52. Eriksson BI, Bauer KA, Lassen MR, Turpie AG. Fondaparinux compared with enoxaparin for the prevention of venous thromboembolism after hip-fracture surgery. *N Engl J Med* 2001; 345(18): 1298-304.

53. Bauer KA, Eriksson BI, Lassen MR, Turpie AG. Fondaparinux compared with enoxaparin for the prevention of venous thromboembolism after elective major knee surgery. *N Engl J Med* 2001; 345(18): 1305-10.

54. Lassen MR, Bauer KA, Eriksson BI, Turpie AG. Postoperative fondaparinux versus preoperative enoxaparin for prevention of venous thromboembolism in elective hip-replacement surgery: a randomised double-blind comparison. *Lancet* 2002; 359(9319): 1715-20.

55. Turpie AG, Bauer KA, Eriksson BI, Lassen MR. Postoperative fondaparinux versus postoperative enoxaparin for prevention of venous thromboembolism after elective hip-replacement surgery: a randomised double-blind trial. *Lancet* 2002; 359(9319): 1721-6.

56. Bergmann JF, Neuhart E. A multicenter randomized double-blind study of enoxaparin compared with unfractionated heparin in the prevention of venous thromboembolic disease in elderly in-patients bedridden for an acute medical illness. The Enoxaparin in Medicine Study Group. *Thromb Haemost* 1996; 76(4): 529-34.

57. Harenberg J, Roebruck P, Heene DL. Subcutaneous low-molecular-weight heparin versus standard heparin and the prevention of thromboembolism in medical inpatients. The Heparin Study in Internal Medicine Group. *Haemostasis* 1996; 26(3): 127-39.

58. Lechler E, Schramm W, Flosbach CW. The venous thrombotic risk in non-surgical patients: epidemiological data and efficacy/safety profile of a low-molecular-weight heparin (enoxaparin). The Prime Study Group. *Haemostasis* 1996; 26 Suppl 2: 49-56.

59. Kleber FX, Witt C, Vogel G, Koppenhagen K, Schomaker U, Flosbach CW. Randomized comparison of enoxaparin with unfractionated heparin for the prevention of venous thromboembolism in medical patients with heart failure or severe respiratory disease. *Am Heart J* 2003; 145(4): 614-21.

60. Harenberg J, Schomaker U, Flosbach CW. Enoxaparin is superior to unfractionated heparin in the prevention of venous thromboembolic events in medical patients at increased thromboembolic risk. *Blood* 1999; 94(Suppl 1): 399a.

61. Cohen AT, Davidson BL, Gallus A, Lassen MR, Tomkowski W, Turpie AG, *et al.* Fondaparinux for the prevention of VTE in acutely ill medical patients [abstract]. *Blood* 2003; 102: 15a.

62. Lacut K, Bressollette L, Le Gal G, Etienne E, De Tinteniac A, Renault A, *et al.* Prevention of venous thrombosis in patients with acute intracerebral hemorrhage. *Neurology* 2005; 65(6): 865-9.

63. Comerota AJ, Katz ML, White JV. Why does prophylaxis with external pneumatic compression for deep vein thrombosis fail? *Am J Surg* 1992; 164(3): 265-8.

64. Cornwell EE, 3rd, Chang D, Velmahos G, Jindal A, Baker D, Phillips J, *et al.* Compliance with sequential compression device prophylaxis in at-risk trauma patients: a prospective analysis. *Am Surg* 2002; 68(5): 470-3.

65. Innohep (package insert). Boulder, CO: Pharmion Corporation, 2003.

66. ARIXTRA (package insert). Research Triangle Park, NC: GlaxoSmithKline, 2004.

67. Lovenox (package insert). Bridgewater, NJ: Aventis Pharmaceuticals, Inc., 2004.

68. Fragmin (package insert). Kalamazoo, MI: Pharmacia & Upjohn Company, 2004.

69. Heparin sodium (package insert). Kalamazoo, MI: Pharmacia & Upjohn Company, 2000.

70. Warfarin sodium (package insert). Pomona, NY: Barr Laboratories, Inc., 2002.

71. Buller HR, Agnelli G, Hull RD, Hyers TM, Prins MH, Raskob GE. Antithrombotic therapy for venous thromboembolic disease: the Seventh ACCP Conference on Antithrombotic and Thrombolytic Therapy. *Chest* 2004; 126(3 Suppl): 401S-428S.

72. Hirsh J, Dalen J, Anderson DR, Poller L, Bussey H, Ansell J, *et al.* Oral anticoagulants: mechanism of action, clinical effectiveness, and optimal therapeutic range. *Chest* 2001; 119(1 Suppl): 8S-21S.

73. Walenga JM, Frenkel EP, Bick RL. Heparin-induced thrombocytopenia, paradoxical thromboembolism, and other adverse effects of heparin-type therapy. *Hematol Oncol Clin North Am* 2003; 17(1): 259-82, viii-ix.

74. Hyers TM. Management of venous thromboembolism: past, present, and future. *Arch Intern Med* 2003; 163(7): 759-68.

75. Merli G, Spiro TE, Olsson CG, Abildgaard U, Davidson BL, Eldor A, *et al.* Subcutaneous enoxaparin once or twice daily compared with intravenous unfractionated heparin for treatment of venous thromboembolic disease. *Ann Intern Med* 2001; 134(3): 191-202.
76. Ginsberg JS. Management of venous thromboembolism. *N Engl J Med* 1996; 335(24): 1816-28.
77. Warkentin TE, Levine MN, Hirsh J, Horsewood P, Roberts RS, Gent M, *et al.* Heparin-induced thrombocytopenia in patients treated with low-molecular-weight heparin or unfractionated heparin. *N Engl J Med* 1995; 332(20): 1330-5.
78. Warkentin TE, Levine M, Hirsh J, Klama LN, Kelton JG. Formation of heparin-induced thrombocytopenia IgG without thrombcytopenia: analysis of a clinical trial (abstract). *Blood* 1995; 86(Suppl 1): 537a.
79. King DJ, Kelton JG. Heparin-associated thrombocytopenia. *Ann Intern Med* 1984; 100(4): 535-40.
80. Silver D, Kapsch DN, Tsoi EK. Heparin-induced thrombocytopenia, thrombosis, and hemorrhage. *Ann Surg* 1983; 198(3): 301-6.
81. Laster J, Cikrit D, Walker N, Silver D. The heparin-induced thrombocytopenia syndrome: an update. *Surgery* 1987; 102(4): 763-70.
82. Martel N, Lee J, Wells PS. Risk of heparin-induced thrombocytopenia with unfractionated and low molecular weight heparin thromboprophylaxis: a meta-analysis. *Blood* 2005; Epub 28 Jun 2005.
83. Hirsh J, Warkentin TE, Raschke R, Granger C, Ohman EM, Dalen JE. Heparin and low-molecular-weight heparin: mechanisms of action, pharmacokinetics, dosing considerations, monitoring, efficacy, and safety. *Chest* 1998; 114(5 Suppl): 489S-510S.
84. von Tempelhoff GF, Harenberg J, Niemann F, Hommel G, Kirkpatrick CJ, Heilmann L. Effect of low molecular weight heparin (Certoparin) versus unfractionated heparin on cancer survival following breast and pelvic cancer surgery: a prospective randomized double-blind trial. *Int J Oncol* 2000; 16(4): 815-24.
85. Green D, Hull RD, Brant R, Pineo GF. Lower mortality in cancer patients treated with low-molecular-weight versus standard heparin. *Lancet* 1992; 339(8807): 1476.
86. Hull RD, Raskob GE, Pineo GF, Green D, Trowbridge AA, Elliott CG, *et al.* Subcutaneous low-molecular-weight heparin compared with continuous intravenous heparin in the treatment of proximal-vein thrombosis. *N Engl J Med* 1992; 326(15): 975-82.
87. Kakkar AK, Levine MN, Kadziola Z, Lemoine NR, Low V, Patel HK, *et al.* Low molecular weight heparin, therapy with dalteparin, and survival in advanced cancer: the fragmin advanced malignancy outcome study (FAMOUS). *J Clin Oncol* 2004; 22(10): 1944-8.
88. Sugiyama T, Itoh M, Ohtawa M, Natsuga T. Study on neutralization of low molecular weight heparin (LHG) by protamine sulfate and its neutralization characteristics. *Thromb Res* 1992; 68(2): 119-29.
89. Bauer KA. Fondaparinux sodium: a selective inhibitor of factor Xa. *Am J Health Syst Pharm* 2001; 58(Suppl 2): 14-17.
90. Weitz JI, Hirsh J, Samama MM. New anticoagulant drugs: the Seventh ACCP Conference on Antithrombotic and Thrombolytic Therapy. *Chest* 2004; 126(3 Suppl): 265S-286S.

91. Dolovich LR, Ginsberg JS, Douketis JD, Holbrook AM, Cheah G. A meta-analysis comparing low-molecular-weight heparins with unfractionated heparin in the treatment of venous thromboembolism: examining some unanswered questions regarding location of treatment, product type, and dosing frequency. *Arch Intern Med* 2000; 160(2): 181-8.

92. Low-molecular-weight heparin in the treatment of patients with venous thromboembolism. The Columbus Investigators. *N Engl J Med* 1997; 337(10): 657-62.

93. Hull RD, Raskob GE, Brant RF, Pineo GF, Elliott G, Stein PD, *et al*. Low-molecular-weight heparin vs heparin in the treatment of patients with pulmonary embolism. American-Canadian Thrombosis Study Group. *Arch Intern Med* 2000; 160(2): 229-36.

94. Simonneau G, Sors H, Charbonnier B, Page Y, Laaban JP, Azarian R, *et al*. A comparison of low-molecular-weight heparin with unfractionated heparin for acute pulmonary embolism. The THESEE Study Group. Tinzaparine ou Heparine Standard: Evaluations dans l'Embolie Pulmonaire. *N Engl J Med* 1997; 337(10): 663-9.

95. de Valk HW, Banga JD, Wester JW, Brouwer CB, van Hessen MW, Meuwissen OJ, *et al*. Comparing subcutaneous danaparoid with intravenous unfractionated heparin for the treatment of venous thromboembolism. A randomized controlled trial. *Ann Intern Med* 1995; 123(1): 1-9.

96. Meyer G, Brenot F, Pacouret G, Simonneau G, Gillet Juvin K, Charbonnier B, *et al*. Subcutaneous low-molecular-weight heparin fragmin versus intravenous unfractionated heparin in the treatment of acute non-massive pulmonary embolism: an open randomized pilot study. *Thromb Haemost* 1995; 74(6): 1432-5.

97. Levine M, Gent M, Hirsh J, Leclerc J, Anderson D, Weitz J, *et al*. A comparison of low-molecular-weight heparin administered primarily at home with unfractionated heparin administered in the hospital for proximal deep-vein thrombosis. *N Engl J Med* 1996; 334(11): 677-81.

98. Koopman MM, Prandoni P, Piovella F, Ockelford PA, Brandjes DP, van der Meer J, *et al*. Treatment of venous thrombosis with intravenous unfractionated heparin administered in the hospital as compared with subcutaneous low-molecular-weight heparin administered at home. The Tasman Study Group. *N Engl J Med* 1996; 334(11): 682-7.

99. Buller HR, Davidson BL, Decousus H, Gallus A, Gent M, Piovella F, *et al*. Fondaparinux or enoxaparin for the initial treatment of symptomatic deep venous thrombosis: a randomized trial. *Ann Intern Med* 2004; 140(11): 867-73.

100. Buller HR, Davidson BL, Decousus H, Gallus A, Gent M, Piovella F, *et al*. Subcutaneous fondaparinux versus intravenous unfractionated heparin in the initial treatment of pulmonary embolism. *N Engl J Med* 2003; 349(18): 1695-702.

101. Lee AY, Levine MN, Baker RI, Bowden C, Kakkar AK, Prins M, *et al*. Low-molecular-weight heparin versus a coumarin for the prevention of recurrent venous thromboembolism in patients with cancer. *N Engl J Med* 2003; 349(2): 146-53.

102. Hull R, Pineo G, Mah A. A randomised trial evaluating long-term low-molecular-weight heparin therapy for three months vs intravenous heparin followed by warfarin sodium in patients with current cancer. *Thromb Haemost* 2003; (suppl): P137a.

103. Horlocker TT, Heit JA. Low molecular weight heparin: biochemistry, pharmacology, perioperative prophylaxis regimens, and guidelines for regional anesthetic management. *Anesth Analg* 1997; 85(4): 874-85.

Chapter 13
Venous reconstruction: indications and success rates

Justin Tan MRCS, *Clinical Research Fellow*
St. Thomas' Hospital, London, UK
Kevin Burnand MS FRCS, *Professor in Surgery*
Head of the Academic Department of Surgery
St. Thomas' Hospital, London, UK

Introduction

Chronic venous insufficiency causes lipodermatosclerosis around the gaiter area of the calf, which is the forerunner of venous ulceration. Primary venous incompetence with reflux is usually the result of vein wall dilatation rather than valvular agenesis or hypoplasia. Secondary valve incompetence and obstruction of the deep veins are invariably the result of a previous thrombosis (post-thrombotic syndrome). In 1958, Palma described the first femoro-femoral cross-over bypass for an iliac vein obstruction and in 1968, Kistner performed the first valve reconstruction for deep vein reflux. Deep venous valvular reconstruction has however, never become popular and the centres performing large numbers of venous reconstructions are very few. The value of venous reconstructive surgery still remains debatable because of a lack of clinical trials. The surgical results are difficult to assess as valve reconstruction or bypasses are almost always performed in combination with superficial vein or perforator vein surgery.

Indications

Patients in whom deep venous surgery can be considered are those with advanced venous insufficiency resulting in ulceration or intractable venous claudication and massive limb swelling, who have failed all forms of conservative treatment e.g. compression stockings or superficial venous surgery. Venous reconstruction is often selected as a procedure of 'last resort' in these patients. Patient selection is vital in achieving reasonable long-term symptomatic improvement. Reconstructive surgery to the deep veins and valve reconstruction should not be considered in the acute phase of venous thrombosis. Other contraindications include a prothrombotic condition (e.g. Lupus, antiphospholipid syndrome, activated protein-C deficiency) or the presence of significant arterial limb ischaemia. When valvular incompetence is being considered, it is important to identify a suitable donor valve e.g. from an arm vein or contralateral saphenous vein. Primary surgical treatment of coexisting incompetence of the superficial and perforating veins, in the absence of major vein obstruction is usually performed before deep vein reconstruction or bypass is considered.

General consideration in deep vein reconstructive surgery

◆ Veins must be handled with care. Excessive traction and crushing causes endothelial damage and invariably predispose to thrombus deposition.

◆ Only atraumatic clamps and the lightest monofilament suture, such as Prolene or PTFE, should be used.

◆ A temporary arteriovenous fistula may be employed to increase venous blood flow in the reconstructed veins in the hope that the risk of thrombosis will be lowered and patency improved.

Venous reconstructive surgery is usually aimed at bypassing the obstructed segment or restoring the valve mechanism. Patients with primary valvular incompetence may have repairable valves which can be managed by direct valvuloplasty, while patients with post-thrombotic legs usually have destroyed valves making direct repair impossible. Valve transposition, transplantation or bypass are the techniques that can be used in the post-thrombotic leg.

Operations for venous incompetence

Internal valve repair (valvuloplasty)

Direct valvuloplasty was first described by Kistner [1]. The most proximal valve in the superficial femoral vein is the one that is most amenable to repair. Alternatively, adjacent valves in the deep femoral and femoral vein may also be repaired. The common femoral, femoral and deep femoral veins are dissected out through a vertical groin incision. The adventitia of the vein must be meticulously dissected out and the valve commissures clearly identified. A marking suture is placed at the apex of the commissure on the anterior surface of the vein to ensure the cusps remain undamaged when the longitudinal venotomy is made. A fine interrupted suture is introduced from out to in on the vein to shorten the leading edge of the redundant cusp to the proper length by plication (Figure 1). It is estimated that by decreasing the valve leaflets by 20% (Figure 1b), this is sufficient to restore competence. In the posterior midline, interrupted sutures are

a   b

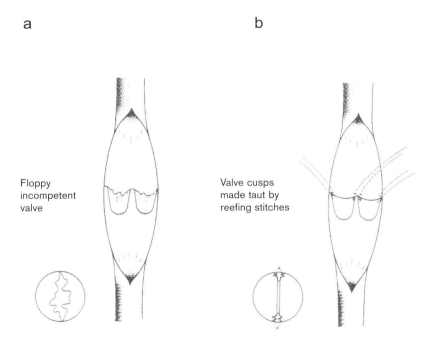

Floppy
incompetent
valve

Valve cusps
made taut by
reefing stitches

Figure 1 Primary valve incompetence corrected by Kistner's direct valvuloplasty. *Reproduced with permission from Edward Arnold. Browse NL, Burnand KG, Irvine AT, Wilson N. Diseases of the Veins. Arnold, 1998.*

introduced at the commissures from the outside to capture both valve cusps. These are passed through the cusps and tied outside the vein to progressively shorten the cusps until they are free of wrinkles and folds. The valve cusps should not be drawn taut. The venotomy is then closed and the valve competence is tested by Harvey's test. Modifications of Kistner's technique have been described and some authors advocate a transverse venotomy to gain access.

Long-term follow-up of valvuloplasty for primary valvular incompetence showed good clinical results in selected patients. Kistner, in an analysis of 4-21 years follow-up, reported clinical improvement of 73% [2] for correction of primary valve incompetence. Postoperative imaging studies correlated well with the clinical outcome; however, physiological studies failed to correlate well with clinical improvement. Few others have reported large series of these procedures which appeared to only affect a small group of patients in Hawaii!

External valve repair

This eliminates the need for venotomy. A series of interrupted sutures are placed on the external surface along the line of the cusp insertion. This produces invagination of the vein wall which narrows the overall circumference restoring valve competence (Figure 2). This technique is quicker and does not require heparin. It requires considerably less dissection than internal repair, but does not produce a precise anatomical repair.

Angioscopic-assisted valvuloplasty

This was first described by Gloviczki [3] in 1991. An angioscope is inserted into a tributary of the great saphenous vein to visualise the incompetent femoral valve cusps as sutures are inserted from the outside to narrow the commissures. The patient must receive a full dose of heparin. The main advantage of this method is that it reduces the operating time, as considerable less dissection is required to insert the angioscope.

a   b   c

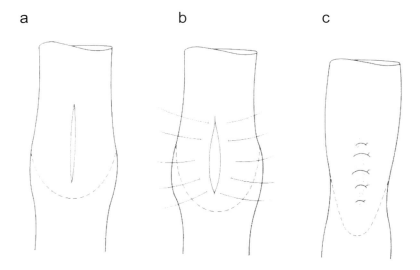

Figure 2 Indirect valvuloplasty by valve plication operation. a) A longitudinal venotomy is made level with the edge of the cusps, midway between the commissures. b) Sutures are placed to close the venotomy, but at an increasing distance from the edge of the venotomy at its centre. c) When the sutures are tied the circumference of the valve ring is reduced. *Reproduced with permission from Edward Arnold. Browse NL, Burnand KG, Irvine AT, Wilson N. Diseases of the Veins. Arnold, 1998.*

External valvular banding

A prosthetic sleeve can be used to externally band a small minority of incompetent valves with reflux secondary to sinus dilatation. A 2-3cm strip made of Dacron, silastic or polytetrafluoroethylene (PTFE) is wrapped around the vein segment containing the valve. This effectively narrows the vein lumen restoring valve competence. The synthetic strip is sutured and then anchored to the adventitia to prevent displacement. A recent innovation based on the same concept is the Venocuff®, which is constructed from a thin reinforced silicone. This can be implanted permanently around a vein at the site of a non-functioning valve. Intraoperatively, the strip test can be used to test competence when the band has been applied.

Valve replacement technique

Psathakis' procedure

In the original operation [4], the gracilis tendon was detached distally and joined across the popliteal fossa to the biceps femoris muscle. Fibrosis and adhesion formation prompted Psathakis to modify his technique. A silastic sling is now sutured to the flexor muscles of the knee and placed around the popliteal vein. When the flexor muscle contracts, as the foot is raised off the ground, the sling tightens around the vein and it is hoped that this prevents reflux. Few others have experience with this operation and it has not been properly assessed in a clinical trial.

Vein transposition

It is possible to insert a competent valve found in either the profunda femoris vein or the upper portion of the great saphenous vein into the venous outflow of patients with popliteal or femoral vein incompetence. A competent valve-bearing segment of the great saphenous vein can be anastomosed (end-to-end), or profunda femoris vein (end-to-side) onto the incompetent femoral vein. It is preferable to anastomose the femoral vein to a competent deep femoral vein rather than the great saphenous to avoid size discrepancy. Arteriovenous fistulae are not usually employed but the patient should be given anticoagulants for three to six months.

Vein transplantation (Taheri procedure)

This is an alternative treatment for femoral or popliteal vein incompetence. A segment of vein containing a valve is taken from the axillary, brachial or even the upper end of the great saphenous vein in the opposite limb. This is usually inserted in the upper popliteal vein. The vein is dissected and a segment is resected before the graft is anatomosed as an interposition graft. Size discrepancy between the donor vein segment and the recipient vein is not critical, as some dilatation of the transplanted vein occurs. Taheri suggested that the graft should be wrapped in Dacron or PTFE mesh to prevent eventual dilatation and later valve incompetence.

Prosthetic valve/xenografts

Other valve replacement techniques have been developed in the last 15 years. The deep vein valves are invariably destroyed by post-thrombotic damage. An autologous vein may not always be available or suitable. The axillary vein may not always contain functioning valves and an 'off-the-shelf' valve is therefore desirable. Initial experiences with implantable prosthetic valves demonstrated a low patency rate. Bio-prostheses [5] incorporating intestinal mucosa have been shown to be effective in animal studies but human studies are awaited.

Xenografts require preservation and neutralisation of antigenic determinants. Glutaraldehyde has been used extensively to treat xenograft valves in the cardiac and arterial circulation but it causes thrombosis in the venous system. There is one report of a glutaraldehyde-preserved bovine monocusp which has been implanted in patients with some success. These authors have argued that they had better results because their techniques preserved the posterior aspect of the patient's vein. Others reported that cryopreserved vein valves became incompetent on thawing, even when a transcommisural valvuloplasty was performed. When implanted, 60% occluded and 70% became incompetent.

Long-term outcome

The risk of postoperative DVT and pulmonary embolism is less than was expected after deep vein reconstruction. The incidence of DVT was found to be as low as 10% in patients with primary deep vein incompetence, although the incidence is higher in post-thrombotic limbs (~20%). Vein transpositions have patencies ranging between 40% and 70%, whereas the patency following transplantation has been between 30%-90%.

Clinical outcomes appear to correlate with the state of valve competence. Many patients whose valves are competent on duplex imaging remain symptomless while patients who develop recurrent symptoms often have occluded veins or malfunctioning valves.

By ten years, patients with primary venous incompetence who have a valve repair (73%) have better outcomes than patients with post-thrombotic syndrome who had valve transposition or transplantation (43%). Two thirds of all patients treated by vein reconstruction are reported to be free of symptoms. Measurements of calf pump function show a modest improvement after valve repair. The clinical improvement always exceeded the improvement in calf pump function.

Operations for deep venous obstruction

The role of deep venous obstruction is probably underestimated, as it is a common feature in the majority of post-thrombotic limbs, often in combination with venous reflux. Surgical intervention may be considered in patients with clear signs of deep venous obstruction and poor collaterals. Cockett's or May-Turner's syndrome, retroperitoneal fibrosis and malignant infiltration of the vena cava are some of the less common causes of deep venous obstruction. Venous bypass surgery should only be considered in those who are debilitated with swelling and venous claudication. Recanalisation of deep vein following acute thrombosis is frequent, so it is prudent to wait at least six to 12 months before contemplating any form of bypass.

Prosthetic iliocaval reconstruction can be performed for unilateral disease when an autologous conduit is not available. Prosthetic bypass can also be considered for occlusions. Externally supported expanded polytetrafluoroethylene (ePTFE) grafts are most often used. The infrarenal IVC is reconstructed with a 16-20mm ePTFE graft, the iliocaval segment usually with a 14mm ePTFE graft and the femorocaval segment with a 10-12mm ePTFE graft. The concomitant construction of a distal temporary femoral arteriovenous fistula is recommended for all prosthetic grafts longer than 10cm to increase flow through the anastomosis and reduce the risk of thrombosis. Short iliocaval bypass across a significant pressure gradient can be performed without an arteriovenous fistula.

Cross venous pubic bypass (Palma-Dale operation)

This is a good bypass for patients with unilateral common or external iliac vein occlusion who do not have significant post-thrombotic damage below the inguinal ligament [6]. Only about 3% of all patients with post-thrombotic damage are suitable candidates for this operation. The great saphenous vein from the opposite limb is divided and mobilised down to the knee before being swung across in a suprapubic tunnel to be anastomosed end-to-end with the common femoral or profunda femoral vein in the groin of the affected limb below the level of the obstruction. The saphenous vein may occasionally be anastomosed to the femoral vein or to the great saphenous vein if this is of good size. An externally supported expanded ePTFE graft of 8mm can be used as a conduit if the contralateral great saphenous vein is inadequate. Prosthetic bypasses are, however, more likely to occlude and should have a temporary arteriovenous fistula constructed to maintain patency. In the largest series of 85 Palma bypasses, 47 of 67 grafts remained patent at the last follow-up that ranged from six months to 15 years. Clinical and functional improvement was achieved in about three quarters of the patients. Expanded PTFE grafts have not performed anything like as well with eight out of nine grafts occluded at an early stage, despite adequate measures.

Saphenopopliteal bypass (May-Husni operation)

This bypass was originally considered for patients with an occlusion of the popliteal or femoral veins. In the original description, the ipsilateral great saphenous vein was rerouted to take flow directly from the popliteal vein and anastomosing it caudal to the site of obstruction. This may be performed by dividing the saphenous vein at the level of the knee and anastomosed end-to-side to the patent distal popliteal vein. An end-to-side arteriovenous fistula can be constructed at the ankle between the posterior tibial artery and one of the paired posterior veins or the saphenous vein just above the medial malleolus. The operation is rarely performed, despite the fact that a functional improvement has been reported in seven different series.

Endovascular treatment

The development of endovascular treatment for iliac vein occlusion has significantly decreased the number of patients who require an open procedure. The initial experience was of balloon dilatation of stenoses in acute iliofemoral thrombosis in patients who had received thrombolytic therapy. Endovascular techniques have now been applied to patients with chronic iliac vein stenoses and occlusions.

Some have advised routine thrombolysis for 24-48 hours to soften thrombus and facilitate the passage of catheters; however, Raju *et al* have performed iliac vein stenting in over 300 cases without any pretreatment thrombolysis or post-treatment anticoagulation with a one-year primary patency rate of 82%. The low pressure venous system is more amenable to balloon dilatation and previously occluded veins can be dilated to 14-16mm. The entire length of the stenosis or occlusion is stented and venous rupture seldom occurs. Stenting of the femoral vein is now recommended to improve inflow and to counteract the effect of immediate venospasm. The flexibility and self-expansion of Wallstents® makes them particularly suitable for venous stenting. They can be accurately placed using intravascular ultrasound (IVUS). Anticoagulation is recommended for six months in almost all cases. As stent technology and design have improved, endovascular intervention has been associated with better patency rates and a reduced need for repeated intervention.

Long-term outcome

Experience with femorocaval or iliocaval bypass is limited and the reported results of surgical treatment for venous obstruction are at best only moderate. In a series of 12 cases, seven grafts were patent at five-year follow-up. At best, open venous reconstruction has a three-year patency of around 50%-60%. Endovascular interventions are best for patients with short, focal lesions, where outcomes are similar to those of stenting iliac disease in the arterial system (70%-90% five-year patency). Major complications such as pulmonary embolism or retroperitoneal haemorrhage are rare (<1%), but early rethrombosis occurs in 10% of patients. Primary and secondary patency rates at two years of 71% and 97% respectively are possible in selected patients with chronic venous occlusion treated endovascularly. Although long-term results of venous stenting are not yet available, initial short and intermediate-term results are encouraging.

Conclusions

Surgical attempts to repair and replace human venous valves have met with mixed success and none of the available techniques is widely accepted. Currently, direct valvuloplasty to restore competence in non-thrombotic deep vein reflux with the correction of coexisting superficial and communicating vein reflux offers the best long-term treatment for calf pump failure. A readily available 'off-the-shelf' valve replacement is not yet available. Improved immunological modification, better biocompatibility and valve preservation technique must be achieved to improve long-term patency rates. Autologous vein bypass is the best method for treating venous obstruction.

Techniques for abolishing reflux in the deep venous system remain the province of the specialist unit. Treatment of coexisting superficial and communicating vein reflux, where appropriate with the provision of good quality graduated compression hosiery, remains central to the management of most patients.

Key Summary

◆ Surgical reconstruction is reserved for patients who suffer from intractable symptoms and have failed all conservative treatments.

◆ Demonstration of significant deep vein reflux by means of investigation is essential prior to surgery.

◆ Internal valvuloplasty is by far the most common type of repair, and good results can be anticipated in about 70% of patients.

◆ The long-term results are better in primary valve incompetence than in post-thrombotic changes.

◆ Endovascular treatment is the first option for symptomatic iliac vein occlusion.

◆ Artificial vein valves are not ready for widespread use.

References

1. Kistner RL. Surgical repair of the incompetent femoral vein valve. *Arch Surg* 1975; 110: 1336-42.
2. Masuda EM, Kistner RL. Long-term results of venous valve reconstruction: a four- to twenty-one-year follow-up. *J Vasc Surg* 1994; 19: 391-403.
3. Gloviczki P, Merrell SW, Bower TC. Femoral vein valve repair under direct vision without venotomy: a modified technique with use of angioscopy. *J Vasc Surg* 1991; 14: 645-8.
4. Psathakis N. [A new operative procedure for the rational treatment of the syndrome of insufficiency of the deep veins of the extremities.]. *Chirurg* 1964; 35: 79-81.
5. Pavcnik D, *et al.* Second-generation percutaneous bioprosthetic valves: a short-term study in sheep. *J Vasc Surg* 2004; 40: 1223-7.
6. Palma EC, Esperon R. Vein transplants and grafts in the surgical treatment of the post-phlebitic syndrome. *J Cardiovasc Surg* (Torino) 1960; 1: 94-107.

Chapter 14
The role of nurse-led clinics

Maxine Taylor BSc (Hons) RGN, *Senior Leg Ulcer Nurse Specialist*
Fiona Slim RGN, *Senior Surgical Care Practitioner*
Cheltenham General Hospital, Cheltenham, UK

Introduction

In recent years, the expansion of nursing roles within the surgical team has been widely accepted. Nurses specialising in key areas such as breast care, stoma management and gastro-intestinal malignancy are now essential members of the surgical team. The New Deal and European Working Time Directive have enforced substantial reductions in the working hours of junior doctors, providing further stimulus for expanded roles for non-medically qualified practitioners [1, 2]. Nurse-led clinics are not a new concept but their number and application have gained momentum in response to patient needs for specialist care and the changing roles in healthcare driven by government initiatives over the last two decades. More recent government initiatives have actively encouraged nurses to respond to patient needs and further enhance their role by taking on a wider range of clinical tasks [3, 4].

Patients with venous disease often have complex ongoing needs, requiring specialist and holistic care. Nurse-led specialist leg ulcer clinics have been implemented in a number of geographical locations in the UK and shown to significantly improve clinical outcomes when compared to traditional models of care [5-7]. This chapter aims to discuss the potential advantages and disadvantages of nurse-led clinics and our experiences of these developments in the vascular unit at Cheltenham.

Nurse-led clinics for venous disease

Advantages

For the patient
Specialist nursing roles can provide greater time for assessment and excellent continuity of care for patients with complex issues such as stoma or breast care. This continuity is essential to develop a rapport between patient and health professional, particularly when the patients are expected to make significant lifestyle changes to comply with treatment. Patients may also perceive nurses as less formal or intimidating and therefore more approachable. This was demonstrated by Vowden [8] who reported improved patient outcomes in clinics where expert nurses were involved in constant and regular leg ulcer management.

For the hospital
Due to imposed limitations on the working hours of doctors, the use of non-medically qualified professionals in specialist healthcare roles has clear advantages for NHS organisations. Expanded nursing roles may alleviate some of the deficiencies left by reduced medical manpower and potentially aid the reduction of outpatient waiting lists and inpatient occupancy, thereby reducing expenses. Permanent specialist nursing posts may also provide greater continuity of care for patients with ongoing healthcare needs and help to facilitate long-term training, audit and research programmes. Venous disease would seem ideally suited to this approach as there are many aspects to the management of patients with venous disease that do not require a doctor. Nurses with the appropriate knowledge and skills, working within clear guidelines and as part of the vascular team, may effectively provide this care.

For the nurse
The introduction of expanded nursing roles signifies evolution from the traditional non-flexible career progression pathways within nursing. The specialist responsibility of these new roles may be associated with increased training and career opportunities, potentially acting as a motivating factor for new nurses entering the profession. This is an

overdue change in a profession associated with low staff retention and poor morale.

Disadvantages

For the patient

The care of patients by non-medically qualified staff may be associated with a reduction in the competence of the practitioner and the quality of care. These roles should therefore be carefully planned and regulated, with the introduction of clear guidelines for training, supervision, assessment of clinical competence and appraisal. Even with appropriate training, the patient's perception may be that the care provided is inferior if their expectations are not met. Moreover, seeing a specialist nurse may not avoid the need to see the medical team, resulting in a greater level of personal inconvenience, due to duplication of care.

For the hospital

The introduction of specialist nurse-led clinics relies heavily on the driving force of lead clinicians and the support of management. Although the introduction of new career opportunities may encourage recruitment into nursing professions in the medium and long term, the current shortage of general nursing staff may be exacerbated in the short term by these roles. There is also a risk that the presence of a specialist nurse may de-skill general nurses from particular aspects of patient care. There may be a level of resentment from general nurses and a reluctance to involve themselves in clinical activities that fall under a specialist nurse role.

For the nurse

The future of specialist nursing roles is uncertain compared to traditional medical roles. Often these roles have developed in an *ad hoc* manner with sporadic funding and may therefore lack a robust career pathway [9, 10]. There is also the potential for competition and conflict between nurse-led services and junior doctor training. Doctors may miss out on exposure to certain patients or procedures, if these patients are assessed and treated away from mainstream clinical areas. The nursing profession may also face a threat from other healthcare workers who could be trained to perform tasks traditionally done by nurses. A blurring of boundaries may lead to a loss of professional identity [11].

Our experiences with nurse-led clinics

Leg ulcer clinic

Background

Prior to 1995, the management of patients with leg ulceration was performed almost exclusively by community nurses. Very few patients underwent any form of vascular assessment, and healing and recurrence rates were poor. Patient treatment was inconsistent and often based on personal preference and tradition rather than clinical evidence. Some patients were referred to the vascular surgical services for secondary care, although no guidelines for referral existed. Following a countywide audit of leg ulcer assessment, healing and recurrence, significant deficiencies in quality of care were identified [7].

In direct response to these audit findings, a specialist nurse-led leg ulcer service was introduced in Gloucestershire in 1995. The service operated under the direct supervision of the Department of Vascular Surgery and aimed to standardise and optimise leg ulcer management across primary and secondary healthcare. Community and hospital-based clinics were introduced and evidence-based management protocols were established. The initial audit was repeated a year after the introduction of the service and demonstrated a significant improvement in outcomes. On the strength of this study and on the recommendation of a countywide working party, the service expanded and has since been accessible to patients throughout Gloucestershire.

Organisation of clinic

Referrals are received from primary and secondary care doctors and nurses and patients themselves. All new patients are invited to a one-stop leg ulcer assessment clinic at one of two District General Hospitals, with the aim of identifying the main aetiological factors for each patient. Evidence-based, protocol-driven treatment is then implemented with regular review in convenient, community-based clinics. All hospital and community clinics are performed by specialist nurses, but in parallel with vascular surgical clinics to allow instant access to medical staff in difficult cases. The management pathway for patients treated by the Gloucestershire leg ulcer service is summarised in Figure 1. After each clinic visit, relevant community nursing teams are contacted to communicate the clinical progress of the patient and any specific changes

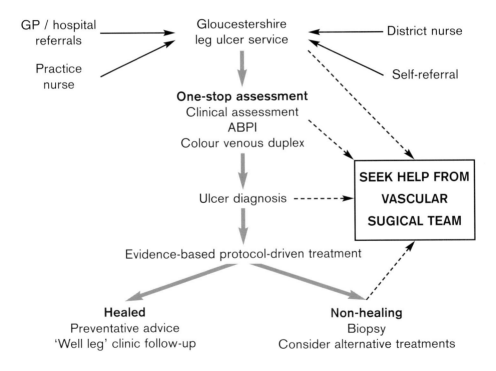

Figure 1 Referral and management pathway for patients treated by the Gloucestershire leg ulcer service.

to management. Patient care carried out between specialist clinic visits is performed by community nurses who can request urgent specialist review if necessary.

The specific responsibilities of the specialist leg ulcer nurses include:

◆ prioritisation and assessment of new referrals;
◆ organisation and interpretation of appropriate investigations;
◆ initiation and monitoring of clinical treatment;
◆ regular review of patients in follow-up clinics based on clinical priority;
◆ recognition of patients requiring further treatment, including arterial procedures and venous surgery;
◆ organisation and running of leg ulcer prevention and health promotion clinics;
◆ carrying out relevant adjunctive procedures including wound biopsy, pinch skin grafting and wound debridement;
◆ communication with hospital services, primary care, patients and relatives;
◆ organisation of local training programmes for community nursing staff;
◆ regular review of clinical care protocols; and
◆ participating in research studies.

Impact of the clinic

The introduction of specialist nurse-led leg ulcer clinics has had a dramatic and positive effect on patient assessment and clinical outcome, in comparison to the previous model of care (Figure 2). As specialist nurses are able to assess, diagnose, treat and review, working within agreed protocols and guidelines, the majority of patients seen in the nurse-led clinics never need to see a doctor.

A rolling programme of leg ulcer study days for community and hospital nurses has been introduced and has helped to increase awareness and skills in the region.

Clinical and outcome details for all patients seen and treated within the Gloucestershire leg ulcer service are recorded prospectively in a

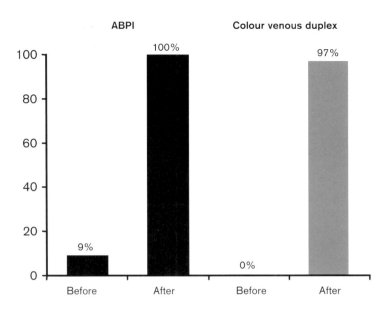

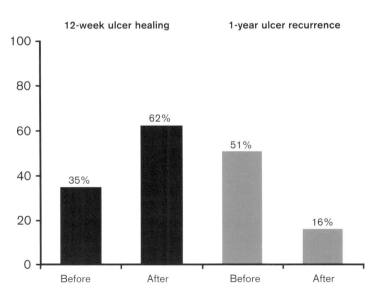

Figure 2 Patient assessment, ulcer healing and recurrence, before and after the introduction of specialist nurse-led leg ulcer clinics.

database, which provides a powerful audit tool for demonstrating clinical and cost-effectiveness.

Varicose vein assessment and follow-up clinics

Background

The assessment of patients with varicose veins and follow-up of patients after venous surgery constitutes a significant proportion of vascular surgical outpatient workload. Patients may present with a wide variety of symptoms and clinical signs, often requiring specialist investigation and treatment to prevent disease progression. The demand for hospital outpatient services is gradually increasing, particularly as there is increasing pressure for surgical teams to accurately audit clinical outcomes following surgery. Moreover, the changes in response to the 'New Deal' for junior doctors and the European Working Time Directive, in some centres, have resulted in increased pressure on already stretched outpatient services.

The reduced presence of junior doctors has led to an inevitable re-allocation of some routine medical duties. New roles such as Surgical Care Practitioners (SCP) have evolved from more traditional nursing positions, with encouragement from the Department of Health and Royal Colleges [12]. SCPs were introduced in Gloucestershire in 2000 and SCP / Nurse Practitioner-led varicose vein clinics were commenced in 2001.

Organisation of clinics

The varicose vein clinics were initially limited to the follow-up of patients after venous surgery. In a similar way to the leg ulcer clinics, all clinics are conducted in parallel to the vascular surgical clinics to ensure that support from the medical team is readily available if needed (Figure 3). During the training process, all patients were seen by both SCP and Consultant Surgeon. Once the SCP was deemed to be competent in the evaluation of patients, direct supervision was discontinued, although support is always immediately available.

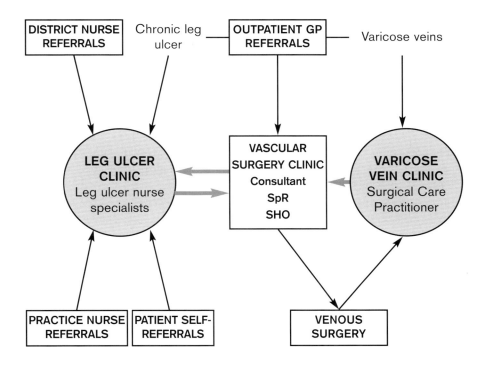

Figure 3 Leg ulcer and varicose vein clinics conducted in parallel with the vascular surgical clinic.

The assessment of patients after varicose vein surgery is performed using a standardised form. The clinical outcome data are then recorded prospectively on a computerised database, which can be readily interrogated to audit complication rates.

Impact of the clinic

Prior to the introduction of varicose vein clinics, local outcomes and complication rates after varicose vein surgery were not audited. In the first three years of the varicose vein clinic, 341 patients were seen and <25% required review by the vascular surgical team. An audit of complication rates for 300 consecutive patients followed-up after varicose vein surgery was performed recently (Table 1). Patients undergoing surgery for recurrent varicose veins were found to have higher rates of wound infection and neurological deficit after surgery. These findings were then incorporated in a patient information leaflet for future patients.

Table 1 Complication rates in 300 consecutive patients followed-up in Surgical Care Practitioner-run varicose vein clinics.

Complication	Incidence after primary varicose vein surgery (n=259)	Incidence after recurrent venous surgery (n=41)
Wound Infection	5%	17%
Numbness	14%	27%
Bleeding	2%	2%
Nerve pain	0%	2%
Other (seroma, MI)	0.4%	2%

Teamwork with medical staff

In our experience, the expansion in nursing roles can be harnessed to increase efficiency within the vascular surgical team. The introduction of nurse-led clinics for venous disease requires dynamic, motivated staff and a period of direct supervision and training which may reduce productivity in the short term. However, with increased experience, we have found that nurse-led clinics become an excellent specialist resource providing high quality care and accurate clinical audit.

Future challenges and prospects

Leg ulcer clinic

Over the last ten years, the number of patients seen by the leg ulcer service has dramatically increased. Healing and recurrence rates have also continued to improve. In 2004, the Government introduced a new system for funding specialist healthcare, known as 'Payment by results'. This has resulted in reviews of leg ulcer clinics by Primary Care Trusts in order to scrutinise spending. It is clear that cost-effectiveness will be increasingly important for specialist leg ulcer clinics to continue to exist. The overall impact of these government reforms is yet to be determined.

Varicose vein clinics

It is hoped that the nurse-led varicose vein clinics will expand to incorporate the routine assessment of new patients referred with varicose veins.

Conclusions

The advent of nurse-led services, whether in response to a pressing need to fill the gaps left by junior doctors, or the desire for advancement of the profession, has changed the way healthcare is organised and enabled a more patient-centred approach. It is now common practice for nurse specialists to be permanent members of vascular surgical teams providing continuity and expertise. Their role in nurse-led clinic services is a natural progression of this.

Key Summary

◆ A specialist nurse-led clinic improves healing and recurrence rates for patients with leg ulceration.

◆ Nurse-led leg ulcer clinics play a pivotal role in co-ordinating care between primary and secondary providers.

◆ Specialist nurses with the necessary skills and knowledge can enhance the vascular team without compromising standards.

◆ SCP-led clinics aid in providing accurate and objective audit.

◆ These extended roles assist in providing quality patient care by improving continuity.

References

1. Department of Health. Junior doctors' hours: the new deal. DoH, London, 1997.
2. British Medical Association. Time's Up: a guide on the EWTD for junior doctors. BMA, 1 August 2004.
3. Department of Health. Making a difference: strengthening the nursing, midwifery and health visiting contribution to health and healthcare. DoH, London, 1999.
4. Department of Health. The NHS Improvement Plan 2004: putting people at the heart of public services. DoH, London, 2004.
5. Murray S. A nurse-led clinic for patients with peripheral vascular disease. *Br J Nurs* 1997; 6: 726-36.
6. Godsell GA. The development of the nurse biopsy role. *Br J Nurs* 2005; 14: 690-2.
7. Ghauri ASK, Taylor M, Deacon JE, Whyman MR, Earnshaw JJ, Heather BP, Poskitt KR. Influence of a specialised leg ulcer service on management and outcome. *Br J Surg* 2000; 87: 1048-56.
8. Vowden KR, Barker A, Vowden MD. Leg ulcer management in a nurse-led hospital-based clinic. *J Wound Care* 1997; 6: 233-6.
9. Humphris D, Masterson A. *Developing new clinical roles: a guide for health professionals.* London: Churchill Livingstone, 2000.
10. Palfreyman S, Trender H. Nurse-led claudication clinics. In: *Pathways of care in vascular surgery.* Beard J, Murray S, Eds. Shrewsbury: Tfm Publishing Ltd., 2002.
11. Cameron A. New role developments in context. In: *Developing new clinical roles: a guide for health professionals.* Humphris D, Masterson A, Eds. London: Churchill Livingstone, 2000.
12. Bulbulia R, Gohel M, Slim F, Whyman M, Poskitt K. Surgical practitioners - current roles and future prospects. In: *Recent advances in surgery,* 27th Ed. Johnson C, Taylor I, Eds. London: Royal Society of Medicine Press Ltd., 2004.

Chapter 15

Venous leg ulcer services: organisation, diagnosis and role of surgery

Manj Gohel MRCS, *Vascular Research Fellow*

Mark Whyman MS FRCS, *Consultant Surgeon*

Keith Poskitt MD FRCS, *Consultant Surgeon*

Cheltenham General Hospital, Cheltenham, UK

Introduction

Chronic venous leg ulceration rarely threatens life or limb, but is extremely common. It causes chronic impairment to patient quality of life [1] and huge financial expense to healthcare providers [2]. Venous hypertension is thought to be primarily responsible for the cutaneous changes that culminate in leg ulceration. Great advances in wound healing research have been made, but a widely accepted mechanism linking venous hypertension and skin damage remains elusive. Despite its clinical importance, leg ulceration is considered an unglamorous and uninteresting condition by many health professionals. Consequently, the management of patients with leg ulceration has largely been left to overworked community nursing teams and the optimum model of care has not been defined.

Multilayer graduated compression therapy is widely considered the gold standard therapy for chronic venous ulceration [3]. Although surgical treatments for venous ulcers have been used for many years, the evidence supporting surgical interventions in this elderly patient population has been limited. Widespread recognition of these deficiencies has stimulated a wave of recent research into optimum models of care and therapeutic strategies.

This chapter aims to discuss models of care for patients with chronic leg ulceration, review the importance of accurate leg ulcer diagnosis and present the evidence for the variety of available surgical interventions.

Organisation of leg ulcer services

Patients with chronic leg ulceration present with a complex pattern of physical, psychological and social morbidities that require a holistic approach to assessment, diagnosis and treatment. In order to meet the complex needs of this population, care of patients should ideally include:

◆ a trained and enthusiastic specialist team with close links to primary care and access to appropriate investigations and hospital specialist services;
◆ detailed clinical assessment to identify aetiological factors;
◆ evidence-based treatment offered at a location convenient for the patient; and
◆ a commitment to the principles of clinical governance with regular appraisal and local audit of clinical outcomes.

For many years, the treatment of patients with leg ulceration has been performed predominantly by community nursing teams. Convenient local treatment provided by familiar faces may be popular with patients. However, this approach may result in incomplete assessment, inconsistent treatment, limited access to secondary care services, inadequate audit and unacceptably poor ulcer healing and recurrence rates [4, 5]. In some geographical areas, patients with ulceration may be referred to vascular surgery teams, although this is likely to be an inefficient use of already stretched services.

In response to these difficulties, a number of centres have developed specialist teams for the assessment and treatment of patients with leg ulceration. In Gloucestershire, a hospital-based specialist nurse-run service was introduced in 1995 operating within the department of vascular surgery. Clinics are held in hospital and community locations. The service supervises the training of local care providers and specialist nurses work closely with community nursing teams ensuring consistent and high quality treatment [4]. This approach allows continuity of care and at the same time, instant access to diagnostic, vascular surgical, dermatological and other specialist hospital services. Similar clinics in Trafford [6], Riverside (Charing Cross) [5] and Sheffield [7] have demonstrated

Table 1 Healing and recurrence rates after introduction of community leg ulcer clinics.

Author	Region	12-week ulcer healing rates		1-year ulcer recurrence rates	
		Without clinics	With clinics	Without clinics	With clinics
Moffatt et al [5] (1992)	Riverside	22%	69%	-	-
Simon et al [6] (1996)	Stockport & Trafford	26%	42%	-	-
Morrell et al [7] (1998)	Sheffield	24%	34%	-	-
Ghauri et al [4] (2000)	Gloucestershire	22%	47%	41%	17%

improved clinical outcomes using this approach (Table 1). Local limitations will inevitably influence the organisation of leg ulcer care, but these studies have demonstrated that the protocol-driven treatment of patients within a specialist setting provides an improved management structure for the treatment of patients with leg ulceration.

Leg ulcer diagnosis

Detailed clinical assessment augmented by appropriate investigations is essential for leg ulcer diagnosis and to identify potentially correctable aetiological factors. In our practice, this is achieved using a one-stop assessment process [8], allowing comprehensive and convenient leg ulcer diagnosis (Figure 1). Measurement of ankle brachial pressure index (ABPI) offers a reliable and reproducible assessment of limb arterial status and should be performed in all patients with leg ulceration. An ABPI >0.85 is considered normal, although patients with an ABPI as low as 0.5 may be safely treated with supervised modified compression bandaging [9]. Falsely elevated ABPI measurements may be seen, especially in diabetic patients, as a result of arterial wall calcification and incompressible vessels. Further arterial assessment may be necessary in some cases.

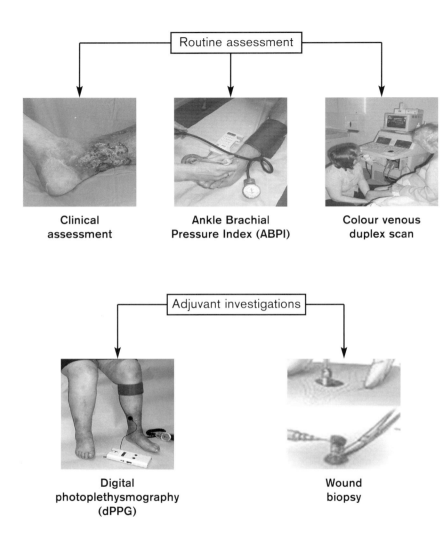

Figure 1 Components of the 'one-stop' assessment for patients with leg ulceration.

Approximately 70% of patients with chronic leg ulceration have a predominantly venous cause (Figure 2), although the definition of a 'venous' ulcer may vary. Traditionally, the presence of venous reflux without arterial compromise was thought to be essential for the diagnosis of a venous ulcer. However, it is clear that venous hypertension may exist even without anatomical evidence of venous reflux, particularly in patients with poor calf muscle pump activity, chronic limb dependency or ankle stiffness [10]. Moreover, the anatomical extent of venous insufficiency correlates poorly with the clinical features of venous hypertension. For these reasons, colour venous duplex scanning is used for the identification of surgically correctable venous disease, not as a diagnostic aid.

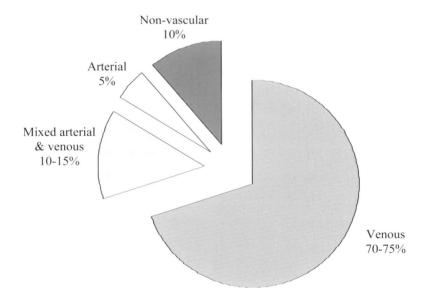

Figure 2 Causes of chronic leg ulceration.

Venous hypertension may be evaluated by assessment of haemodynamic and pressure changes in ulcerated legs. Invasive pressure monitoring uses a cannulated foot vein attached to a pressure transducer and is considered the gold standard in venous haemodynamic investigation. A simpler and less invasive test is digital photoplethysmography (PPG), which uses light reflectivity to estimate venous pressure changes based on skin capillary engorgement. As haemodynamic assessment usually requires repetitive movements of the foot, this may not be possible in patients with ankle stiffness. Invasive pressure monitoring may provide a useful measurement of functional venous disease, but its use is generally limited to research activities or in exceptional clinical cases. The use of PPG with a tourniquet may be useful identifying those patients with mixed superficial and segmental venous reflux who may benefit from superficial venous surgery. Finally, as malignancy may be present in 1-2% of chronic ulcers, wounds with a suspicious appearance or no evidence of healing after three months should undergo biopsy.

The role of surgery for leg ulceration

Numerous surgical interventions have been proposed for the treatment of chronic leg ulceration. In our experience, procedures to improve arterial circulation are necessary only in a minority of cases, as patients with moderate arterial compromise can be safely treated with supervised modified compression therapy [9].

For patients with venous ulceration, treatment strategies aim to reduce chronic venous hypertension. The mainstay of treatment for venous ulceration is below-knee multilayer compression graduated from 40mmHg at the ankle to 17-20mmHg at the upper calf [3]. However, surgical interventions may also have a role in reducing venous hypertension.

Surgical correction of venous reflux

Chronic venous hypertension secondary to venous reflux in the leg is accepted as the major cause of venous ulceration. Deep venous damage causing either reflux or obstruction was traditionally thought to be of greatest importance, although in recent years, superficial venous reflux has been confirmed to be a significant cause of primary venous ulceration. Calf perforator incompetence without reflux in other veins is uncommon, representing less than 3% of all cases (Figure 3). Correction of refluxing superficial venous segments would seem a logical strategy to eliminate venous hypertension in this patient group and a number of approaches have been forwarded.

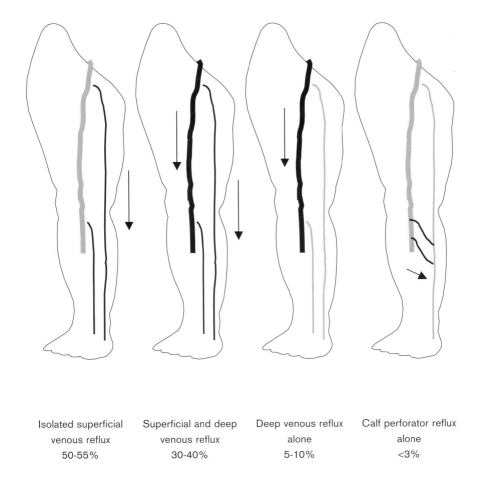

| Isolated superficial venous reflux 50-55% | Superficial and deep venous reflux 30-40% | Deep venous reflux alone 5-10% | Calf perforator reflux alone <3% |

Figure 3 Patterns of venous reflux in patients with chronic leg ulceration.

Superficial venous surgery

Operations to disconnect saphenofemoral and / or saphenopopliteal junctions with stripping of the great saphenous vein to the knee are established as acceptable treatments for varicose veins in the distributions of great and small saphenous veins. The widespread use of such procedures in patients with venous ulceration has been restricted, possibly as a result of the erroneous beliefs that the majority of patients had deep reflux and superficial venous surgery may be detrimental. Prior to the widespread use of compression therapy, some studies showed that surgery may improve venous ulcer healing [11]. However, the recent ESCHAR randomised study compared the effect of surgery and compression with compression alone in chronic venous ulceration. This study confirmed the findings of previous non-randomised work and concluded that adding superficial venous surgery to compression did not affect ulcer healing, but significantly reduced ulcer recurrence at one and three years [12, 13]. This benefit was greatest for patients without deep venous reflux (Figure 4), although reduced recurrence for some patients with coexistent superficial and deep venous reflux was seen.

Despite superficial venous surgery, a number of patients still suffer recurrent ulceration, suggesting that the benefits of adjuvant surgery may be greater in some cases. This may be related to recurrence of superficial venous incompetence or incomplete procedures. Identification of those most likely to benefit from superficial venous surgery is desirable, particularly as this cohort of patients is often elderly and frail and many patients potentially suitable for surgery are unfit or unwilling for operative intervention. In our experience, limb haemodynamic assessment using digital photoplethysmography (dPPG) with a below-knee tourniquet to mimic superficial venous surgery may predict the haemodynamic improvement after surgery [14] and potentially identify those patients likely to derive most benefit from operative intervention (unpublished data). A proposed algorithm for surgical treatment is presented in Figure 5. Further clarification of the relevance of venous investigations may help avoid unnecessary procedures and further refine the role of surgery in these patients.

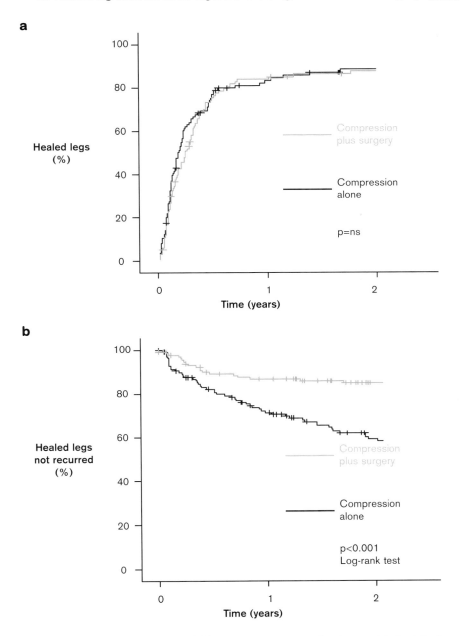

Figure 4 a) Ulcer healing and b) recurrence rates for legs with isolated superficial reflux treated with compression alone, or compression with superficial venous surgery (ESCHAR trial) [13].

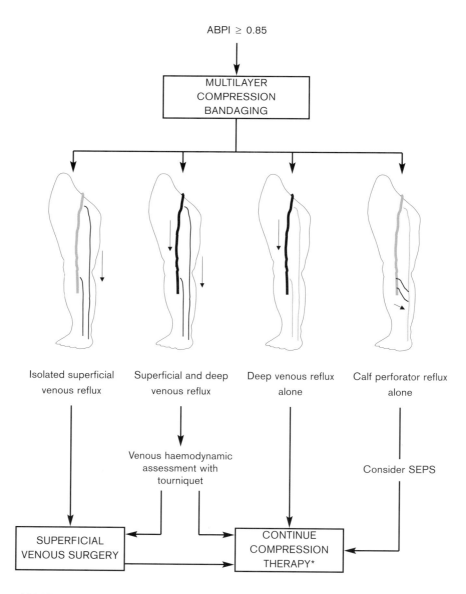

ABPI ≥ 0.85

MULTILAYER
COMPRESSION
BANDAGING

Isolated superficial
venous reflux

Superficial and deep
venous reflux

Deep venous reflux
alone

Calf perforator reflux
alone

Venous haemodynamic
assessment with
tourniquet

Consider SEPS

SUPERFICIAL
VENOUS SURGERY

CONTINUE
COMPRESSION
THERAPY*

* Multilayer graduated bandaging for open ulcers and class II elastic stockings for healed legs.

Figure 5 Proposed algorithm for surgical treatment of patients with chronic venous ulceration.

Perforator surgery

Incompetent calf perforating veins are seen in >50% of patients with chronic leg ulceration, although their importance is a subject of continuing controversy. Open approaches to calf perforator vein ligation have been largely replaced by the minimally invasive Subfascial Endoscopic Perforator Surgery (SEPS), which is popular in the USA and parts of Europe. However, in the studies that reported favourable results following SEPS, most patients were also treated with superficial venous surgery. Some calf perforating veins may be avulsed during traditional saphenous surgery, although this is generally not documented or assessed. Moreover, some studies have suggested that flow from deep to superficial veins may not be pathological in all cases and may be reversed after standard saphenous surgery. These concerns have meant that SEPS is rarely performed in the UK and is usually considered only for the small group of patients with isolated perforator vein incompetence.

Surgery for deep venous reflux

Various procedures attempting to restore competence to refluxing deep venous segments have been described. These include venous valvuloplasty, venous bypass and prosthetic valve transplants. However, the literature supporting the use of these procedures is limited and a recent Cochrane review concluded that there was insufficient evidence to recommend the use of deep venous surgery to correct reflux [15].

Foam sclerotherapy, VNUS and endovenous laser

A variety of new techniques to obliterate superficial venous reflux are gaining credence. These include foam sclerotherapy and other catheter-based procedures, although the evidence for their use in venous ulceration is limited. Elderly patients with chronic venous ulceration are often unfit or unwilling to undergo open surgery. These interventions are appealing options as they may be performed in the outpatient setting using local anaesthesia and are less invasive than traditional surgery. Whether these alternatives are as effective as traditional superficial venous surgery in reducing venous hypertension remains unproven. Even if foam sclerotherapy, VNUS and endovenous laser therapy are less effective than superficial venous surgery, there may be adequate haemodynamic and clinical benefit for these techniques to be useful treatment options in the elderly leg ulcer population. Clinical studies are currently in progress and may help clarify these issues.

Skin grafting

The use of skin grafting to improve the healing rate of non-healing venous ulcers has been proposed by a number of authors. Grafts are commonly used to cover a variety of dermal defects with favourable clinical outcomes and may be applied in a number of ways. Autografts harvested from the thigh are common and may be performed on an outpatient basis by trained specialist nurses. Although the use of grafting has been evaluated in a number of studies, prospective randomised trials are rare and the use of grafts is usually guided by the personal experience and preference of individual clinicians.

Wound debridement

It is generally accepted that clean wounds, with a granulating bed are more receptive to skin grafting. Wound debridement to remove slough may be necessary and numerous agents for removal of necrotic tissue have been used. Debridement strategies include dry dressings, aggressive irrigation, surgery, hydrogels and enzyme therapy. Debridement using larval therapy (maggots) is well tolerated, effective and our technique of choice in wounds with excessive slough. However, level 1 evidence is generally lacking and a recent systematic review of debridement in chronic wounds concluded that further studies including cost-effectiveness analyses were needed [16].

Pinch skin grafting

Small areas of skin may be harvested from the thigh of patients using local anaesthetic and applied to the surface of large, clean venous ulcers. The aim is to provide epithelial islands on an ulcer from where further healing can progress (Figure 6). Although few prospective studies have investigated the benefits of pinch skin grafting in addition to compression, a randomised trial showed a 12-week healing rate of 74% which was significantly greater than patients treated with porcine dermis [17]. Centres

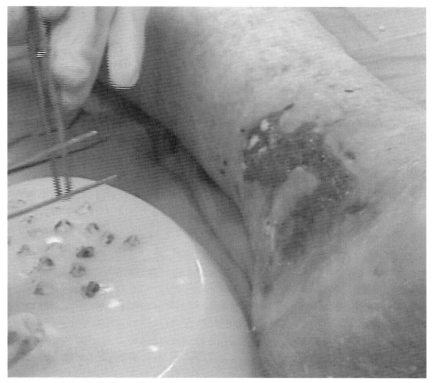

Figure 6 Pinch skin grafting for venous ulceration.

that routinely using pinch skin grafting have also reported favourable results [18], but further randomised trials are needed. In our practice, pinch skin grafts are performed by nurse specialists on an outpatient basis and utilised for ulcers >3cm in diameter with a granulating base.

Split skin grafts

Split skin grafts include the epidermis and part of the dermis and may be harvested using a dermatome. These grafts may be meshed and therefore have the advantage of being suitable for large areas of ulceration, while allowing wound exudate to escape. However, donor sites may be painful, prone to infection and slow to heal. A Cochrane review investigated the role of skin grafting in venous ulceration and concluded that insufficient evidence was available to assess the effectiveness of split or pinch skin grafting [19]. Further studies are needed to clarify if skin grafts offer additional benefit over and above compression therapy and if so, which grafting technique is best.

Skin substitutes

In recent years, a number of substitute skin products for use in chronic wounds have been introduced. Artificial skin such as Dermagraft™ (Smith & Nephew, Hull, UK) is cultured from neonatal foreskin and contains fibroblasts, extra-cellular matrix components and other cells necessary for growth factor release and tissue healing. A systematic review concluded that bioengineered skin products may improve healing when used with compression [19], but the products evaluated are not currently available in the UK and some have been withdrawn in the USA. Despite the undoubted potential of skin substitutes, they are expensive and the available evidence is insufficient to support their routine use in patients with venous ulceration.

Conclusions

The management of patients with chronic venous ulceration has seen dramatic improvements in recent years. Recent research has highlighted the importance of multilayer compression therapy and experiences from numerous centres have shown that patients are best treated by specialist leg ulcer teams in dedicated clinics that have close links with primary and secondary care. Superficial venous surgery has also been identified as an important adjunct to leg ulcer management by reducing venous ulcer recurrence rates, although surgery is often unpopular or refused. The introduction of new, less invasive techniques to correct superficial venous incompetence may improve the uptake of venous procedures in this elderly patient group.

Skin grafting using pinch skin, split skin or artificial skin substitutes may have a role in the management of large or non-healing wounds, although further trials are needed. Despite advances in therapy, non-healing ulcers are common and are an ongoing clinical challenge. Further research is essential to develop effective treatment strategies for these patients.

Key Summary

◆ Leg ulcer care should be provided by specialist teams with links to community and secondary care.

◆ Ulcer diagnosis may be aided using a one-stop assessment.

◆ Superficial venous surgery in addition to compression reduces venous ulcer recurrence in some patients.

◆ There is insufficient evidence to support the routine use of skin grafting.

References

1. Phillips T, Stanton B, Provan A, Lew R. A study of the impact of leg ulcers on quality of life: financial, social and psychological implications. *J Am Acad Dermatol* 1994; 31: 49-53.

2. Nelzen O. Leg ulcers: economic aspects. *Phlebology* 2000; 15: 110-4.

3. Cullum N, Nelson EA, Fletcher AW, Sheldon TA. Compression bandages and stockings for venous leg ulcers. *Cochrane Database of Systematic Reviews* 2000; CD000265.

4. Ghauri ASK, Taylor M, Deacon JE, Whyman MR, Earnshaw JJ, Heather BP, Poskitt KR. Influence of a specialized leg ulcer service on management and outcome. *Br J Surg* 2000; 87: 1048-56.

5. Moffatt CJ, Franks PJ, Oldroyd M, Bosanquet N, Brown P, Greenhalgh RM, McCollum CM. Community clinics for leg ulcers and impact on healing. *Br Med J* 1992; 305: 1389-92.

6. Simon DA, Freak L, Kinsella A, Walsh J, Lane C, Groarke L, McCollum C. Community leg ulcer clinics: a comparative study in two health authorities. *Br Med J* 1996; 312: 1648-51.

7. Morrell CJ, Walters SJ, Dixon S, Collins KA, Brereton LML, Peters J, Brooker CGD. Cost effectiveness of community leg ulcer clinics: randomised controlled trial. *Br Med J* 1998; 316: 1487-91.

8.   Ghauri ASK, Currie IC, Grabs AJ, Whyman MR, Farndon JR, Poskitt KR. Improving the diagnosis of chronic leg ulcers: a one-stop vascular assessment clinic in a community service. *Phlebology* 1998; 13: 148-52.

9.   Ghauri ASK, Nyamekye I, Grabs AJ, Farndon AJ, Poskitt KR. The diagnosis and management of mixed arterial/venous leg ulcers in community-based clinics. *Eur J Vasc Endovasc Surg* 1998; 16: 350-5.

10.   Barwell JR, Taylor M, Deacon J, Davies C, Whyman MR, Poskitt KR. Ankle motility is a risk factor for healing of chronic venous leg ulcers. *Phlebology* 2001; 16: 38-40.

11.   Bello M, Scriven M, Hartshorne T, Bell PR, Naylor AR, London NJ. Role of superficial venous surgery in the treatment of venous ulceration. *Br J Surg* 1999; 86: 755-9.

12.   Barwell JR, Davies CE, Deacon J, Earnshaw JJ, Esher J, Heather BP, Mitchell DC, Taylor M, Whyman MR, Poskitt KR. Comparison of surgery and compression with compression alone in chronic venous ulceration (ESCHAR study): randomised controlled trial. *Lancet* 2004; 363: 1854-9.

13.   Gohel MS, Barwell JR, Taylor M, Chant T, Earnshaw JJ, Heather BP, Mitchell DC, Whyman MR, Poskitt KR. Superficial venous surgery reduces venous ulcer recurrence - 3-year results from the ESCHAR trial. *Br J Surg* 2005; 92: 506.

14.   Sullivan JG, Ghauri ASK, Whyman MR, Poskitt KR. Preoperative digital photoplethysmography predicts improvement in venous function after superficial venous surgery for chronically ulcerated limbs. *Phlebology* 1998; 13: 142-7.

15.   Abida A, Hardy SC. Surgery for deep venous incompetence (Cochrane Review). *The Cochrane Library*, 2000.

16.   Bradley M, Cullum N, Sheldon T. The debridement of chronic wounds: a systematic review. *Health Technology Assessment* 1999; 3(17): 1-90.

17.   Poskitt KR, *et al.* Pinch skin grafting or porcine dermis in venous ulcers: a randomised clinical trial. *Br Med J (Clin Res Ed)* 1987; 294: 674-6.

18.   Oien RF, Hansen BU, Hakansson A. Pinch grafting of leg ulcers in primary care. *Acta Derm Venereol* 1998; 78: 438-9.

19.   Jones JE, Nelson EA. Skin grafting for venous leg ulcers. *The Cochrane Database of Systematic Reviews* 2000; Issue 2. Art. No.: CD001737. DOI: 10.1002/14651858. CD001737.pub2.

Chapter 16

Deep vein thrombosis and travel

John H Scurr BSc MB BS FRCS

Consultant Surgeon, The Lister Hospital, London, UK

Introduction

A number of anecdotal reports have linked deep vein thrombosis with flying. In 1954, Homans described three cases of deep vein thrombosis (DVT) following flights [1]. Throughout the 1960s there were a number of reports emanating from hospitals in close proximity to airports suggesting passengers who had flown long distances were at increased risk of developing thrombo-embolic complications. The first prospective study published in the *Lancet* in 2001 showed a relatively high incidence of symptomless deep vein thrombosis in passengers who had completed long haul flights [2]. Since that time a number of studies have shown symptomatic DVTs occurring in between 1% and 3% of passengers undertaking long journeys [3]. Although the problem has been specifically related to air travel it would appear that the problem is linked to immobility and that all travellers, including travellers by bus, train and car, are equally at risk [4]. The term 'economy class syndrome' was coined by Symington and Stack [5]. This group wrongly attributed venous thrombosis to cramped conditions. We know from more recent studies that all passengers, whatever class, are at risk of developing deep vein thrombosis. The risk seems to be related to the duration of travel, the frequency of travel and the interval between episodes. The diagnosis of deep vein thrombosis is notoriously unreliable. Less than 50% of patients with a deep vein thrombosis will develop symptoms and many patients developing the classic symptoms of a swollen tender calf will have another cause. In many instances a deep vein thrombosis is a transient event with the body's own fibrinolytic system removing the clot. It is only in passengers where the clot extends or embolises that significant problems arise.

Retrospective clinical studies of people suffering from thromboembolism suggested up to 20% to have taken some form of long haul travel in the preceding month. Conflicting results have appeared in the literature with Ferrari *et al* [4] reporting an association with travel for greater than four hours increasing the risk of DVT, and Kraaijenhagen and colleagues [6] suggesting that travel within the previous four weeks with travelling times of up to five hours did not increase the risk of deep vein thrombosis. When Kraaijenhagen's results were reanalysed, passengers who had travelled for more than 12 hours did have a significant increase in the incidence of deep vein thrombosis.

It is probable that with better techniques for diagnosing deep vein thrombosis, such as duplex ultrasound imaging, that the true incidence of deep vein thrombosis in the general population is considerably greater than was originally thought. Deep vein thrombosis may well represent a transient episode with thrombus occurring during periods of immobility and disappearing as soon as mobility is restored. It is only in patients where the immobility persists or there are other underlying risk factors that the deep vein thrombosis becomes clinically significant and may then give rise to a pulmonary embolus.

There is no doubt that a link between travel and deep vein thrombosis exists. It is probable that in most cases more than one factor is required before somebody will develop a venous thrombosis. Much of the work associated on risk factors and development of deep vein thrombosis has been done in hospital-based patients [7]. We know for example that age is an important risk factor. Concurrent medical conditions, a past history of thrombo-embolic disease, recent surgery/trauma and an underlying thrombophilia are very important risk factors. Any combination of these associated with prolonged immobility is likely to lead to the development of deep vein thrombosis. In the majority of cases, many factors are involved in the episode of venous thrombosis and this would certainly explain why people who travel regularly with no problems suddenly experience difficulties. In very young patients the existence of a thrombophilia may explain the occurrence of deep vein thrombosis, with 7-

10% of the population suffering from a genetically acquired thrombophilia. It is therefore perhaps not surprising that we see deep vein thrombosis in younger patients.

The 'economy class syndrome' does not exist. This was an unfortunate name for a condition which affects all travellers. For the same reason we should discard 'flight-related thrombosis' and replace this with 'traveller's thrombosis', expecting people travelling by all means of transport to be at risk.

Latest developments in traveller's thrombosis

In October 2000 the House of Lords published a report recognising an association between travel and deep vein thrombosis [8]. The report also highlighted the need for further research. The lack of properly controlled randomised studies, epidemiological studies and a general reluctance by all areas of the travel industry to investigate, has left a number of questions unanswered.

Prior to October 2000, the Civil Aviation Authority regulated aircraft and aircrew. There was no specific regulatory body looking after the interests of passengers, although ultimate responsibility for these passengers lay with the Department of Transport. Following a series of consultations it was agreed that the Civil Aviation Authority would take responsibility for passengers, and a separate department was set up within the CAA to monitor and advise on passenger health. Whilst this department addresses issues relating to flight-related deep vein thrombosis, one must not lose sight of the fact that many travellers by bus, by boat or train will also experience similar problems.

In 2001, Scurr *et al* studied 200 patients with no previous history of venous thrombo-embolic complications, all travelling for more than eight hours and returning within three weeks of their departure [2]. The incidence of deep vein thrombosis was detected using duplex ultrasound imaging, patients being scanned before and after travel. Half the patients were randomly allocated to wear graduated compression stockings. Given that anti-embolism stockings are effective in supine patients they chose to use Class II graduated compression stockings producing 20mmHg compression at the ankle. Below-knee stockings were used for the purpose of this study. In the non-stocking group the incidence of duplex ultrasound-detected DVT was 10%. In the stocking group no DVTs were detected, but four cases of superficial thrombophlebitis in patients with prominent varicose veins were noted.

A study by Bendz *et al*[9] looking at people exposed to hypobaric hypoxia suggested an increase in clotting factors. A similar study repeated under the auspices of the WHO failed to demonstrate any changes in thrombosis-related indicators in patients who sustained hypobaric hypoxaemia for a duration of eight hours. Currently, the only link between travel and the development of DVT is immobility. There does not appear to be any specific link related to travelling in an aeroplane other than immobility and the fact that aeroplanes today can travel for much greater periods of time.

A number of risk factors are associated with the development of deep vein thrombosis, and these were clearly established when studying patients who were entering hospital to undergo surgery [7]. These risks include age, past history of thrombo-embolic complications, concurrent illnesses, history of disseminated malignancy and thrombophilia.

Any traveller with significant risk factors should receive advice and prophylaxis. Effective methods of prophylaxis, again derived from our experience treating hospitalised patients, include mechanical methods of prophylaxis, graduated compression stockings and intermittent pneumatic compression, and chemical methods of prophylaxis including low-molecular-weight heparin. Intermittent pneumatic compression is cumbersome and therefore unlikely to have a place until the units are reduced in size. We have demonstrated that foot exercise devices, the Airwalker and the Airogym, do promote the flow of blood through the deep veins [10]. Exercising against resistance produces a very much more effective flow through the deep veins than simply moving the feet in a circular manner. Although we now have good data that it promotes the flow of blood, no studies have yet been carried out to show that this exercise or the promotion of blood through the deep veins actually reduces the incidence of deep vein thrombosis. We know from studies carried out using elastic compression stockings, again in hospitalised patients, that the prevention of venous distension is as important as the overall increase in blood flow in the reduction of deep vein thrombosis.

The use of aspirin remains controversial. The evidence that aspirin is effective in preventing venous thrombosis is limited. Aspirin is associated with significant gastro-intestinal bleeding complications. Everybody has stopped short of recommending aspirin as a routine method of DVT prophylaxis for travellers, because of the potential risks of bleeding [11]. Alternative preparations are currently being investigated. Zinopin® (a food supplement with antiplatelet properties) , a combination of French maritime pine bark and ginger, has been shown to reduce not only deep vein thrombosis, but superficial thrombophlebitis in travellers [12]. In a recent open study, passengers taking Zinopin® were noted to have reduced ankle oedema and a reduction in cramps during travel [13]. A large double blind, placebo controlled study is currently underway to confirm the efficacy of Zinopin®.

In terms of prophylaxis, all passengers who have significant risk factors should receive prophylaxis. Those passengers embarking upon long haul flights with no risk factors should be encouraged to take plenty of exercise before, during, and after travel, to avoid drinking too much alcohol, and to avoid taking any medication which causes drowsiness and therefore increasing immobility. The use of graduated compression stockings and/or Zinopin® offers benefits both in terms of ankle swelling and in terms of preventing superficial vein problems.

Conclusions

The ability to travel further and more frequently has led to an increased awareness in traveller's thrombosis. Traveller's thrombosis is related to prolonged immobility. Common risk factors including age, concurrent illness, a past history of thrombo-embolic disease and thrombophilia can be identified and prophylaxis applied. For the majority of travellers the risk is small, but sensible advice about mobility, the use of graduated compression stockings, and Zinopin® is recommended. The true incidence of venous thrombo-embolism during travel is only now being recognised because of advances in diagnostic methods. With better epidemiological data, controlled studies can now be carried out to see if we can influence the incidence of this problem.

Key Summary

◆   The true incidence of traveller's thrombosis remains unknown.

◆   Traveller's thrombosis is related to immobility.

◆   All travellers, not just those in the air, are at risk.

◆   Travellers should undergo risk assessment and those with identifiable risk factors should receive prophylaxis.

◆   For most travellers the risk is small, but simple precautions such as mobility, compression stockings, and/or Zinopin®, are recommended.

References

1.   Homans J. Thrombosis of the deep leg veins due to prolonged sitting. *N Engl J Med* 1954; 250: 148-9.
2.   Scurr JH, Machin SJ, Bailey-King S, Mackie IJ, McDonald S, Smith PD. Frequency and prevention of symptomless deep vein thrombosis in long-haul flights: a randomised trial. *Lancet* 2001; 357: 1485-9.
3.   Belcaro G, Geroulakos G, Nicolaides AN, Myers KA, Winford M. Venous thromboembolism from air travel: the LONFLIT study. *Angiology* 2001; 52: 369-74.
4.   Ferrari E, Chevallier T, Chapelier A, Baudouy M. Travel is a risk factor for venous thromboembolic disease: a case-control study. *Chest* 1999; 115: 440-4.
5.   Symington IS, Stack BHR. Pulmonary thromboembolism after travel. *Br J Chest* 1977; 17: 138-40.
6.   Kraaijenhagen RA, Haverkamp D, Koopman MMW, Prandoni P, Piovella F, Büller H. Travel and the risk of venous thrombosis. *Lancet* 2000; 356: 1492-3.
7.   THRIFT Consensus Group. Risk of and prophylaxis for venous thromboembolism in hospital patients. Thromboembolic Risk Factors. *Br Med J* 1992; 305: 567-74.
8.   House of Lords: Science and Technology Committee. Air Travel and Health. 2000. www.parliament.the-stationery-office.co.uk/pa/ld199900/ldselect/ldsctech /121/12101.htm.

9.   Bendz B, Rostrup M, Sevre K, Anderson T, Sandset PM. Association between acute hypobaric hypoxia and activation of coagulation in human beings. *Lancet* 2000; 356: 1657-8.

10. Coleridge Smith P. Effect of exercise using the Airogym on femoral vein flow velocity. www.airogym.com/trails.php.

11. Geerts WH, Pineo GF, Heit JA, Bergqvist D, Lassen MR, Colwell CW, Ray JG. Prevention of venous thromboembolism: the seventh ACCP conference on antithrombotic and thrombolytic therapy. *Chest* 2004; 126(3 Suppl): 338S-400S.

12. Scurr JH, Gulati OP. Zinopin - the rationale for its use as a food supplement in traveller's thrombosis and motion sickness. *Phytother Res* 2004; 18(9): 687-95.

13. Scurr JH, Gulati OP. Zinopin - its use as a food supplement in traveller's thrombosis, oedema and motion sickness. *European Bulletin of Drug Research* 2005; 13: 77-81.

Chapter 17

Foam sclerotherapy

Philip Coleridge Smith DM FRCS

Reader in Surgery, UCL Medical School, London, UK

Introduction

Sclerotherapy has been used to treat varicose veins for 150 years. Many authors have published their techniques and results but only a few are mentioned here for brevity. A more detailed review of the history of this subject has been published recently [1]. One of the first descriptions of a method of sclerotherapy that resembles the techniques used today was published in a monograph by Dr. R. Thornhill in 1929 [2]. The apparatus used to make the injections included a syringe which had been modified to include a small glass window between the syringe and the needle. This was used to aspirate blood from the vein to be injected in order to confirm that the tip of the needle was in the lumen of the vein. Thornhill used a solution of quinine and urethane to treat veins.

Fegan devised his own injection-compression technique which involved firm bandaging of the lower limb following injection of a sclerosant [3]. This method, along with strategies described by other European authors, has been widely used for more than half a century. In the UK and other northern European countries, sclerotherapy is substantially less popular than in southern European countries such as France, Spain and Italy. The reasons for this are not entirely clear but there was a diminishing interest in sclerotherapy in the UK following the publication of a randomised study between sclerotherapy and surgery published by Hobbs in 1984 [4]. This showed that the outcome of surgical treatment after ten years was substantially better than conventional sclerotherapy. Many took this to mean that sclerotherapy was not a very useful treatment in the management of varicose veins and its use declined in the UK and northern European countries.

Ultrasound-guided sclerotherapy

In the 1980s ultrasound was introduced for the diagnosis of venous disease of the lower limb. In France, where enthusiasm for the use of sclerotherapy had remained strong, this led Schadeck and Vin to improve the efficacy of their treatment by using ultrasound imaging to guide the placing of injections into incompetent saphenous trunks [5, 6]. This method of treatment was found to achieve obliteration of the saphenous trunks in a substantial proportion of patients, resulting in long-term relief from varices. As with conventional sclerotherapy, the problem of recanalisation of veins was encountered in up to one quarter of patients at one year [7]. Proponents of sclerotherapy argue that even if recurrence occurs the resulting varices and incompetent saphenous trunk are easily managed by further sessions of sclerotherapy.

Foam sclerotherapy - the origins

In 1944, Orbach described the 'air block' technique. A small volume of air is included in the syringe with the sclerosant. The air is injected ahead of the sclerosant in order to prevent blood diluting the sclerosant and reducing its efficacy. In 1950, Orbach published a further paper describing the use of a foam which he created by vigorously shaking a syringe containing air and sclerosant to produce a froth [8]. He modestly records that this method was also suggested by Foote [9]. Fegan refers to the use of sodium tetradecyl suphate (STS) as a foam in the management of vulval varices of pregnancy in his book on sclerotherapy, originally published in 1967 [10].

The next significant advance came in 1993 when Cabrera suggested that foam could be created using carbon dioxide mixed with a polidocanol, a detergent sclerosant [11]. Cabrera published a further article in 1997 describing his experience in 261 limbs with long saphenous varices and eight patients with vascular malformations [12]. He had used sclerotherapy with foam, guiding his injections by ultrasound imaging. Some of the varicose veins reached 20mm in diameter. He considered that foam greatly extended the range of vein sizes which could be managed by sclerotherapy. He felt that the increased efficacy of foam was attributable to it displacing blood from the treated vein and increasing the contact time between the sclerosant and the vein. He used a 'microfoam', that is a foam made of very small bubbles, which was created by the use of a small rotating brush.

How is foam made?

A series of authors has described methods of preparing 'home-made' foam which may be used for ultrasound-guided sclerotherapy. Monfreux described a method necessitating a glass syringe that produced small quantities of polidocanol foam which he used in a series of patients with truncal varicose veins [13]. Sadoun described a method of preparing foam using a plastic syringe avoiding the need for reusable glass syringes [14]. Subsequently, Tessari has described a method of preparing foam using two disposable syringes and a three-way tap [15]. This method can be used to produce large quantities of foam suitable for treating saphenous trunks and large varices. Frullini has added his own method of producing foam to this increasing list [16] based on that of Flückinger [17].

The most widely used method is that of Tessari which is readily achieved using materials available in most clinics (Figure 1). Two syringes are connected using a 3-way tap. These can be either 2ml or 5ml syringes or a combination. A mixture of sclerosant and air is drawn into one syringe at a ratio of one part of sclerosant to three or four parts of air. This author usually uses 0.5ml of sclerosant and 1.5ml of air to produce 2ml of foam. The sclerosant can be STS 1-3% (Fibrovein, STD Pharmaceuticals, Hereford, UK) or polidocanol 0.5-3% (Sclerovein, Resinag AG, Zurich, CH). Low concentrations of polidocanol (0.5%) make better foam when mixed 1:1 with air. The mixture is oscillated vigorously between the two syringes about ten or 20 times. The tap can be turned slightly to reduce the aperture and increase the smoothness of the foam. The foam produced in this way is stable for about two minutes so it should be injected immediately it has been created. The use of 2ml aliquots of foam encourages the use of smaller overall volumes of foam.

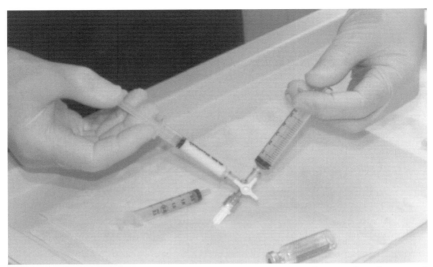

Figure 1 Tessari's method of creating sclerosant foam. A mixture of sclerosant (3% Fibrovein) and air is oscillated between two syringes connected by a 3-way tap.

How is the foam used?

Sclerosant foam can simply be used instead of liquid sclerosant in the management of varicose veins and reticular varices not associated with truncal saphenous incompetence. I suggest that nothing stronger than 1% STS foam is injected into saphenous varices and 0.5% polidocanol into reticular varices, since stronger concentrations may cause thrombophlebitis and encourage skin pigmentation over injected veins. The advantage of using foam in these veins is that more varices appear to be treated per injection and lower volumes of sclerosant are required. Since veins injected with foam have blood displaced from them and develop a spasm it is usually obvious which veins have been treated without the need for ultrasound imaging.

A technique for treating saphenous trunks

Foam sclerotherapy, as described by Cabrera, was intended to be used to treat saphenous trunks as an alternative to surgery. This requires ultrasound-guided injection, since the saphenous trunks cannot be readily treated safely and effectively without imaging control. Cabrera described cannulation of the affected saphenous trunk followed by injection of foam until the vein has been completely filled along with its tributaries. Any unfilled tributaries were managed by injection using a butterfly needle. Other strategies are possible and it is common practice in France to inject the saphenous trunk using a needle and syringe. The complete length of the incompetent vein and tributaries are managed by several injections, carried out over a number of sessions. Direct needle injection has the advantage of simplicity but in some regions, such as the popliteal fossa, a number of large arteries may lie adjacent to the small saphenous vein. Inadvertent intra-arterial injection causes disastrous results and therefore it is recommended that injection of saphenous trunks is carried out through an intravenous catheter or butterfly, which facilitates checks to ensure that the intended vein is injected. Therefore, anyone carrying out this treatment should be familiar with the ultrasound anatomy of the lower limb veins and have gained competence at foam injection under the guidance of an experienced sclerotherapist.

It may be tempting simply to inject the foam into a large tributary of the saphenous vein, but in the author's experience this strategy does not work! It is essential that the saphenous trunk is filled with sclerosant foam without contamination from blood arriving from any source. Blood appears to inhibit the effect of foam, so even a large tributary joining the saphenous trunk proximal to the level of the injection may allow the vein above this level to remain patent, even though foam reached the vein (Figure 2). In treating the great saphenous vein (GSV) I usually place an 18g IV cannula at the level of the knee or just above, and then search for any large tributary (>3mm in diameter) which joins the saphenous trunk proximal to this level and inject the tributary with 2ml of foam before commencing work on the saphenous trunk. If it is decided to treat the GSV in the calf as well, a 23g butterfly is placed in this vein 10-15cm below the knee. When treating the small saphenous vein (SSV) the cannula is placed 10-15cm below the popliteal skin crease and the butterfly in the distal half of the calf (Figure 3).

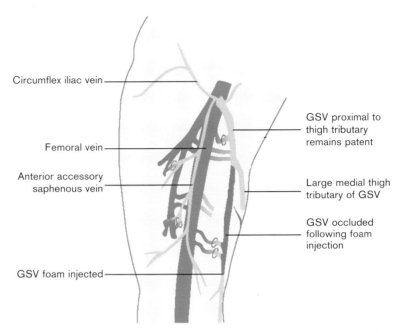

Circumflex iliac vein

GSV proximal to thigh tributary remains patent

Femoral vein

Anterior accessory saphenous vein

Large medial thigh tributary of GSV

GSV occluded following foam injection

GSV foam injected

Figure 2 Foam treatment of the saphenous vein in the thigh: a large medial thigh tributary of the GSV carries sufficient blood to the saphenous trunk to prevent obliteration of the proximal part of the vein.

All cannulas and butterflies are placed in the limb with the patient recumbent, lying on one or other side, to facilitate access to the saphenous trunk to be treated. There is no need to place the limb in the dependent position to facilitate cannulation, although some practitioners use a tourniquet placed proximally on the limb to increase the size of veins.

It is important to check that the needle or cannula is correctly placed. It should be possible to aspirate dark venous blood from the vein. Injection of 0.9% saline under ultrasound monitoring is used to confirm that the solution enters the intended vein and does not extravasate.

If there are any varices that need treating in the first session these are injected before commencing work on the saphenous trunks. The limb is then elevated to empty the veins, resting it in a simple sling attached to a drip pole (Figure 4). I start with the most distally placed cannula or butterfly

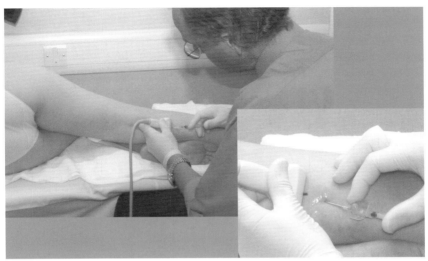

Figure 3 Ultrasound-guided cannulation of the SSV. The patient lies supine on her left side. Local anaesthetic is injected and an 18g IV cannula is introduced 10-15cm distal to the saphenopopliteal junction (SPJ).

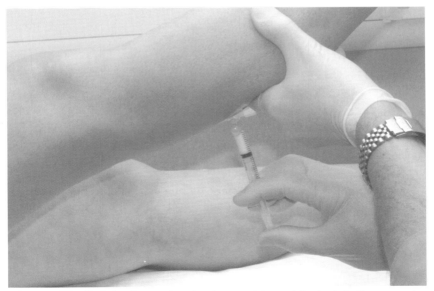

Figure 4 The limb is elevated and sclerosant foam injected via the cannula.

and inject 1% Fibrovein or polidocanol foam in the calf. In the GSV in the thigh and in the proximal SSV, 3% Fibrovein is injected to maximise the effect in the most important regions.

A wide range of accounts of different volumes of foam that should be injected are reported. Cabrera injected up to 100ml of his foam, whereas other authors have averaged 1-2ml in a single session. This author's usual practice is to inject 6-8ml of foam into the GSV in the thigh and about 4ml in the calf. In the SSV, 6ml is injected proximally and 2ml distally, injecting 2ml at a time, with a pause of half to one minute between injections. This allows the treated vein to go into spasm and maximises the contact time between the injected foam and the vein. It also slows the rate of entry of foam into the main veins. Cabrera described compression at the saphenofemoral junction (SFJ) and SPJ to minimise this, but it is inevitable that foam will reach the deep veins. I promote mixing of the foam with the blood in the deep veins by asking the patient to perform active dorsiflexions at the ankle. This strategy has minimised the number of occasions on which thrombosis has spread from superficial veins to the muscle veins of the calf.

Following completion of a session of treatment, firm compression bandaging is applied. Sclerotherapists usually employ a short stretch or limited stretch bandage rather than an elastic stocking (Figure 5). The latter readily allows veins to expand and is ineffective at preventing thrombophlebitis. The time for which bandaging should be applied has not been established by any scientific work. Fegan recommended uninterrupted compression for six weeks, but in the author's experience, the most patients will tolerate is 1-2 weeks.

At subsequent sessions the extent of occluded veins is established by duplex ultrasonography. Unoccluded sections of saphenous trunk are re-treated along with all residual varices. Further bandaging is applied over the treated regions. If thrombus distends superficial saphenous varices or trunks, then this is aspirated under ultrasound control using a suitably large needle inserted under local anaesthetic. This strategy is also effective should post-sclerotherapy thrombophlebitis develop.

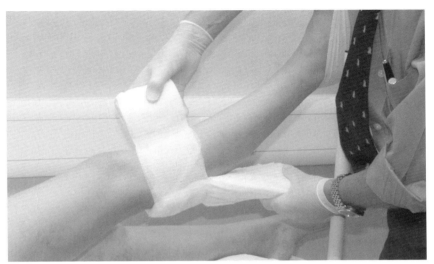

Figure 5 A compression bandage is applied below the knee. PehaHaft (Hartmann, Germany) is applied over Velband to compress the SSV and varices arising from it.

In the author's experience one or two sessions of treatment are required to treat one leg completely. If both legs are treated in the same course of treatment then three sessions are usually required, although more may be necessary if extensive varices are present.

Appropriate patients to treat by foam sclerotherapy

The patients who are the easiest to treat are those with primary GSV or SSV varices, where the saphenous trunk is 5-8mm diameter. The vein is easy to cannulate and the varices are not usually too extensive. Smaller veins take a little practice in cannulation and larger veins are associated with more extensive varices. Experts in ultrasound-guided injection commonly treat veins in the range 0.5-1mm in diameter. Recurrent varices are more complex since they are often not straight, unless there is a residual saphenous trunk. Cannulation is therefore a little more difficult. However, ultrasound-guided injection of these veins is much less complex than recurrent varicose vein surgery and as effective as injecting primary incompetent saphenous trunks.

The question as to which patients are the most suitable for this type of treatment depends on a number of factors, not least the patient's expectations. Those with modest sized saphenous trunks and varices of limited extent are ideal and can often be managed in a single session if only one limb is affected. Some patients have a mortal fear of hospitals and anaesthesia, and are happy to agree to anything that will avoid this. Elderly patients and those with leg ulcers often fall into this group and are pleased to have avoided surgical intervention. Even those with very large or extensive varices may be treated without apparent disadvantage [18], although more sessions may be required. I have managed a small number of patients with ultrasound evidence of previous deep vein thrombosis using foam sclerotherapy. In this group, as with surgery, a five-day course of low-molecular-weight heparin at prophylactic doses is given. No DVT has been seen in these patients.

Few patients are unsuitable for foam sclerotherapy. Those who are very anxious or needle-phobic are probably best managed surgically. I occasionally decline to treat very elderly or frail patients or those with severe concurrent medical conditions. Where treatment for varicose veins is clinically indicated, e.g. for bleeding or ulceration, foam sclerotherapy is the least invasive intervention in frail patients.

Complications

Complications arising from foam sclerotherapy are those which may also arise from and have been previously described in connection with conventional liquid sclerotherapy. Problems may arise locally at the site of injection, in the same limb or systemically.

Local complications include extravasation of sclerosant foam associated with skin necrosis. This is more commonly seen with STS than with polidocanol foam, which is much less likely to cause problems if it leaks from a vein during treatment.

Thrombophlebitis occurs reasonably frequently following sclerotherapy but is readily managed by aspiration of thrombus. Frullini reported two cases of skin necrosis and seven of thrombophlebitis in a series of 196 patients treated by foam sclerotherapy.

Deep vein thrombosis may occur following surgery or sclerotherapy for varicose veins. Gastrocnemius veins in the calf are at risk of exposure to sclerosant foam injected into superficial varices. Frullini also reported one case of gastrocnemius thrombosis and a further case of popliteal vein thrombosis in his series of 196 patients. I have suggested a strategy above in order to minimise the risks of this complication.

Systemic complications which have been described following both liquid and foam sclerotherapy include visual disturbance and chest symptoms, including coughing. These occur in about 1-2% of patients. Visual disturbance often occurs in patients with a previous history of migraine associated with a visual aura. They develop a scotoma following treatment, which resolves completely within 30-60 minutes. There is some evidence that this may be attributable to the passage of bubbles via a patent foramen ovale (PFO), which is in any case present in 10-20% of people. There is a rapidly expanding literature on the association of PFO and migraine in the general population [19]. These effects resolve spontaneously without sequelae and can by minimised in patients where they have occurred previously, in my experience, by ensuring that the patient lies supine for 20-30 minutes following treatment.

Severe allergic reactions to sclerosants are rare but not unknown. These represent the most severe adverse reaction to treatment. Anyone performing sclerotherapy of any type should be suitably equipped to deal with such an event.

Outcomes

Cabrera has published a clinical series of 500 lower limbs treated by foam sclerotherapy. He reported that after three or more years 81% of treated great saphenous trunks remained occluded and 97% of superficial varices had disappeared. This required one session of sclerotherapy in 86% of patients, two in 11% and three sessions in 3% of patients. No DVT or pulmonary embolism was encountered in this series. Frullini and Cavezzi have reported similar data in a series of 453 patients [20]. Early observations showed that 93% of veins remained occluded after treatment with Tessari foam.

No randomised study of foam sclerotherapy in comparison to surgery has yet been published, although a multicentre European study has been conducted. Studies of this type are necessary to evaluate the real differences between these methods of treatment.

Reticular varices and saphenous varices

Foam sclerotherapy has also been investigated in the management of small varices, including reticular veins and telangiectases. In 1999, Henriet reported his results in 10,000 patients with reticular varices and telangiectases of the lower limb treated between the years 1995-8 [21]. He found that the outcome of foam treatment in small varices was excellent and that reduced volumes and concentrations of sclerosant could be employed compared to liquid sclerosants. Benigni reported the findings of a pilot study comparing liquid and foam sclerosants. He measured the outcome using a visual analogue scale to describe the improvement in appearance. He found that foam resulted in a 20% improved appearance compared to liquid sclerosant [22].

Conclusions

Foam sclerotherapy offers an alternative to surgical intervention for patients with varicose veins. It can be conducted on an outpatient basis and is far less complex than endovenous laser therapy or radiofrequency ablation of saphenous veins. It can also be used in primary or recurrent truncal incompetence as well as in tributaries and small varices. The longevity of this treatment has yet to be established in comparison to surgery. Ultrasound imaging studies suggest that 85-90% of veins treated in this way remain occluded after three years. This is comparable to endovenous laser therapy and radiofrequency ablation, and provides similar rates of neovascularisation as reported following surgery. This technique promises to be a useful addition to the methods currently in use for managing superficial venous incompetence.

Key Summary

◆ Foam sclerotherapy is widely used in many countries for the management of superficial venous incompetence.

◆ Treatment is directed initially towards incompetent saphenous trunks which are injected under ultrasound control. Residual varices and saphenous tributaries are then treated.

◆ This treatment is painless, in contrast to surgery, endovenous laser therapy or radiofrequency closure, which facilitates outpatient treatment. No complex equipment is required other than an ultrasound imaging machine resulting in low costs in comparison to surgical management. Patients can normally continue their usual work following treatment.

◆ Complications include skin necrosis due to the sclerosant, thrombophlebitis and deep vein thrombosis. Occasionally, transient visual disturbance and chest problems may also arise. Peripheral nerves are not at risk during this treatment.

◆ Primary or recurrent saphenous trunks, tributaries and varices, as well as reticular varices, may be managed by foam sclerotherapy.

◆ Published clinical series suggest that 85-90% of treated saphenous trunks remain occluded three years following treatment.

References

1. Wollmann JC. The history of sclerosing foams. *Dermatol Surg* 2004; 30: 694-703.
2. Thornhill R. *Varicose veins and their treatment by 'empty vein' injection.* London: Balliere, Tindall & Cox, 1929: 64.
3. Fegan WG. Injection with compression as a treatment for varicose veins. *Proc R Soc Med* 1965; 58: 874-6.
4. Hobbs JT. Surgery or sclerotherapy for varicose veins: 10-year results of a random trial. In: *Superficial and deep venous diseases of the lower limbs.* Tesi M, Dormandy JA, Eds. Turin: Panminerva Medica, 1984: 243-8.
5. Schadeck M, Allaert F. Echotomographie de la sclérose. *Phlébologie* 1991; 44: 111-30.
6. Vin F. Echo-sclérothérapie de la veine saphène externe. *Phlébologie* 1991; 44: 79-84.
7. Kanter A, Thibault P. Dermatol saphenofemoral incompetence treated by ultrasound-guided sclerotherapy. *Surg* 1996; 22: 648-52.
8. Orbach EJ. The thrombogenic activity of foam of a synthetic anionic detergent (sodium tetradecyl sulfate NNR). *Angiology* 1950; 1: 237-43.
9. Foote RR. *Varicose veins.* London: Butterworth & Co, 1949: 1-225.
10. Fegan G. *Varicose veins: compression sclerotherapy.* London: Heinemann Medical, 1967: 1-114.
11. Cabrera Garido JR, Cabrera Garcia-Olmedo JR, Garcia-Olmedo Dominguez MA. Nuevo meodo de esclerosis en las varices tronculares. *Pathologia Vasculares* 1993; 1: 55-72.
12. Cabrera Garrido JR, Cabrera Garcia-Olmedo JR, Garcia-Olmedo Dominguez MA. Elargissement des limites de la schlérothérapie: noveaux produits sclérosants *Phlébologie* 1997; 50: 181-8.
13. Monfreux A. Traitement sclérosant des troncs saphènies et leurs collatérales de gros calibre par le méthode mus. *Phlébologie* 1997; 50: 351-3.
14. Sadoun S, Benigni JP. The treatment of varicosities and telangiectases with TDS and Lauromacrogol foam. XIII World Congress of Flebology, 1998, Abstract Book, p 327.
15. Tessari L. Nouvelle technique d'obtention de la scléro-mousse. *Phlébologie* 2000; 53: 129.
16. Frullini A. New technique in producing sclerosing foam in a disposable syringe. *Derm Surg* 2000; 26: 705-6.
17. Flückinger P. Nicht-operative retrograde Varizenverödung mit Varsylschaum. *Schweizer Med Wochenschrift* 1956; 86: 1368-70.
18. Barrett JM, Allen B, Ockelford A, Goldman MP. Microfoam ultrasound-guided sclerotherapy treatment for varicose veins in a subgroup with diameters at the junction of 10mm or greater compared with a subgroup of less than 10mm. *Dermatol Surg* 2004; 30: 1386-90.
19. Holmes DR Jr. Strokes and holes and headaches: are they a package deal? *Lancet* 2004; 364: 1840-2.
20. Frullini A, Cavezzi A. Sclerosing foam in the treatment of varicose veins and telangiectases: history and analysis of safety and complications. *Dermatol Surg* 2002; 28: 11-5.
21. Henriet JP. Expérience durant trois années de la mousse de polidocanol dans le traitement des varices réticulaires et des varicosités. *Phlébologie* 1999; 52: 277-82.
22. Benigni JP, Sadoun S, Thirion V, Sica M, Demagny A, Chahim M. Télangiectasies et varices réticulaires traitement par la mousse d'aetoxisclérol à 0.25% présentation d'une étude pilote. *Phlébologie* 1999; 52: 283-90.